APPLIED STATISTICS IN HEALTH SCIENCES

APPLIED STATISTICS IN HEALTH SCIENCES

SECOND EDITION

NSN RAO

MSc, PhD, FAMS, FIPHA
Ex-Reader of Biostatistics &
Co-ordinator of Health Projects (Professor Grade)
Banaras Hindu University, Varanasi
Hon. Professor of Biostatistics
RFPG College for Psycho-Social
Rehabilitation, Bengaluru
Visiting Professor
Institute of Health Management Research, Bengaluru
Ex Team Leader, Technical Support Unit
United Nations Population Fund, New Delhi

NS MURTHY

MSc, PhD, FAMS, FSMS
Ex-Deputy Director (Senior Grade)
Institute of Cytology and Preventive Oncology (ICMR)
Emeritus Medical Scientist
Indian Council of Medical Research
New Delhi

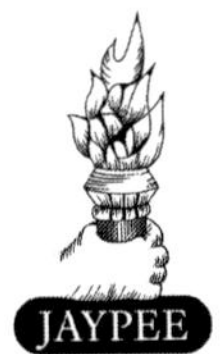

JAYPEE BROTHERS MEDICAL PUBLISHERS
The Health Sciences Publisher
New Delhi | London

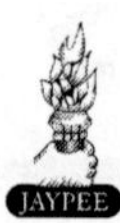

Jaypee Brothers Medical Publishers (P) Ltd

Headquarters
EMCA House
23/23-B, Ansari Road, Daryaganj
New Delhi 110 002, India
Landline: +91-11-23272143, +91-11-23272703
+91-11-23282021, +91-11-23245672
E-mail: jaypee@jaypeebrothers.com

Corporate Office
4838/24, Ansari Road, Daryaganj
New Delhi 110 002, India
Phone: +91-11-43574357
Fax: +91-11-43574314
E-mail: jaypee@jaypeebrothers.com

Overseas Office
J.P. Medical Ltd
83 Victoria Street, London
SW1H 0HW (UK)
Phone: +44 20 3170 8910
E-mail: info@jpmedpub.com

EU GPSR Authorised Representative
Logos Europe, 9 rue Nicolas Poussin
17000, La Rochelle, France
Phone: +33 (0) 6 67 93 73 78
E-mail: contact@logoseurope.eu

Website: www.jaypeebrothers.com
Website: www.jaypeedigital.com

North America Office
1745, Pheasant Run Drive, Maryland Heights (Missouri), MO 63043, USA Ph: 001-636-6279734
e-mail: jaypee@jaypeebrothers.com, anjulav@jaypeebrothers.com

Central America Office
Jaypee-Highlights Medical Publishers Inc., City of Knowledge, Bld. 237, Clayton, Panama City, Panama Ph: 507-317-0160

Applied Statistics in Health Sciences

First Edition: **2008**
Second Edition: **2010**
Reprint: **2026**

ISBN 978-81-8448-801-2

Typeset at JPBMP typesetting unit
Printed at: Samrat Offset Pvt. Ltd.

Preface to the Second Edition

We are thankful to all the research workers, teachers and students for the overwhelming response extended to the first edition of this book. Copies of the first edition of the book were exhausted in a span of one year. It gives us immense pleasure to place the second edition of the book before all the research workers. Even though not many changes have been incorporated in this edition, due to short span of time between the first edition and the present one, there are certain minor modifications done in the light of the feedback received from the users of the book.

We firmly believe that there is every scope for improvement and we earnestly solicit for suggestions for improvement in further editions of this book.

We are grateful to all the users of this book and expect a similar response for the present edition.

NSN Rao
NS Murthy

Preface to the First Edition

Importance of application of statistical methodologies in Health Sciences could hardly be disputed. Though Statistical Methodologies were used mostly in Epidemiological studies in the past, the application of the subject has been widely recognised in all branches of Health Sciences. However, the application of Statistical Methodologies in Health Sciences has been hamstrung in the absence of a simple and standard book with proper illustrations from the field of Health Sciences.

In this context, 'Elements of Health Statistics' which was brought out by the Senior author way back in 1978, was very well received by the students, teachers and research workers in Health Sciences. Over the past four decades, the authors have been engaged in teaching and guiding research workers of different deciplines in health sciences and were prompted to enlarge the scope of the book keeping in view of the needs in Health Science Research. The experiences gained by the authors have been utilised in formulating different chapters in the book. Various chapters included in the present book cover most of the routine aspects of application of Research methods and Statistics useful in different deciplines of Health Sciences. In view of the fact that workers engaged in Health Science research are deficient in mathematical aspects, even elementary calculations are not ignored in presenting the examples.

Authors are sure that this book will meet the routine needs of all research workers in Health Sciences.

Many students, friends and colleagues have given many useful suggestions in enlarging the scope of the present book. Their contributions are highly acknowledged.

NSN Rao
NS Murthy

Contents

1 Chapter Statistics and Research

Meaning of Statistics

The word statistics usually conveys to a lay man an impression about numerical facts. But to a scientific worker it means the methodology of collection, compilation and interpretation of numerical facts. The numerical facts, which one comes across in health or biological sciences, such as, pulse rate, haemoglobin percentage level, number of births and deaths taking place in a year etc., are all affected and controlled to a large extent by a number of factors—biological, environmental, social and so on. Hence, whenever the meaning of certain numerical figures are to be understood and their cause and effect in terms of different factors is to be elicited, certain analytical procedures are to be followed. In order that these numerical facts convey certain useful meaning, they are to be collected in a scientific manner. The methodology of such collection and meaningful interpretation of numerical facts is known as "Statistics". In broader sense, the science of Statistics deals with the methodologies of collection of numerical facts as well as with the analysis of variability present in the observation and also subjecting the factual descriptions to objective tests to validate their reliability.

The principles of Statistical Methodology are same in whichever branch of Science they are applied. However different nomenclatures are adopted depending upon the usage and application in different fields of Science. Mainly a medical professional or a bioscientist is interested in the following branches.

(i) *Biostatistics*: This branch deals with the methodologies of collection, elucidation and interpretation of numerical facts relating to the biological sciences. Medical Statistics is a part of this broader science.

(ii) *Health Statistics*: This branch in particular deals with the methodology of collection, compilation and interpretation of numerical facts concerned with the health and ill health of the human population. Some of these are births, diseases or deaths in the background of various factors controlling them. However, when numerical facts dealing with only births, deaths, marriages, divorces, etc. are considered, the branch of statistics is known as *'Vital Statistics'*. Some people used to call Vital Statistics as the *'Book Keeping'* of the humanity and the present day Health Statistics has developed out of these Vital Statistical methods. This subject, in fact, is a branch of wider science known as "Demography" which deals with the study of human population.

Statistical Methodologies play an important role in research. Before going through these methodologies it is apt to understand some concepts of research.

Meaning and Characteristics of Research

Research is a careful investigation or inquiry, especially through scientific methods, aimed at searching new facts or verification of established facts under various situations, in any branch of knowledge. Scientific research is a systematic and objective attempt to provide answers to certain questions. The purpose of research is to discover and develop an organised body of knowledge through application of scientific procedures.

Numerous definitions are available of the term "Research". The appropriate definition would be, "an honest, exhaustive, intelligent searching for facts and their implications with reference to a given problem, which may lead to development of theories, concepts, generalisations and principles". The ultimate outcome of any research should be to define authentic and verifiable knowledge leading to definite contributions in the field studied.

Thus all research should generally aim at gaining new knowledge emphasising on the general principles, investigated in a systematic and accurate manner through valid procedures of data collection, analysis and interpretation. Research is characterised by the following considerations:

i. Research is always directed towards the solution of a problem. In other words, in research, the researcher always tries to answer a question or relate two or more variables under study.

ii. Research is always based upon empirical or observable evidence. It implies that research is related basically to one or more aspects of a real situation and deals with concrete data that provides a basis for external validity of research results. The researcher rejects those principles or revelations, which are subjective and accepts only those revelations or principles, which can be objectively observed.

iii. Research involves precise observation and accurate description. The researcher selects reliable and valid instruments to be used in the collection of data and uses some statistical measures for accurate description of the results obtained.

iv. Research gives emphasis to the development of theories, principles and generalisations, which are very helpful in accurate prediction regarding the variables under study. On the basis of the sample observed and studied, the researcher tries to make sound generalisations regarding the whole population. Thus, research goes beyond immediate situations, objects or groups being investigated by formulating generalised statements or theory about these factors.

v. Research is characterised by systematic, objective and logical procedures. The researcher tries to eliminate his bias and makes every possible effort to ensure objectivity in the methods employed, data collected and conclusion reached. He frames an objective and scientific design for the smooth conduct of his research. He also makes a logical examination of the procedures employed in conducting his research work so that he may be able to check the validity of the conclusions drawn. The research procedures adopted should confirm to the accepted scientific and systematic methods and should be free from personal biases or prejudice and should be capable of being verified. All cause and effect for a particular phenomenon should be substantiated with evidence.

vi. Research is marked by patience, courage and unhurried activities. Whenever the researcher is confronted with difficult questions, he must not answer them hurriedly. He must have patience and courage to think over the problem and find out the correct solution.

vii. Research requires that the researcher has full expertise of the problem being studied. He must know all the relevant facts regarding the problem and must review the important literature associated with the problem. He must also be aware of sophisticated statistical methods of analysing the obtained data.

viii. Research is replicable. The designs, procedures and results of scientific research should be replicable so that any person other than the researcher himself may assess their validity. Thus, one researcher may use or transmit the results obtained by another researcher. Thus, the procedures and results of the research are replicable as well as transmittable.

ix. Research pre-supposes ethical neutrality. It aims at making only adequate and correct statements about population under study and confirms to various ethical norms .

x. Research uses probabilistic predictions. The predictions made out of the observations confirm to the existing probability of occurrence of events under observation.

xi. Finally, research requires skill of writing and producing the report. The researcher must know how to write the report of his research. He must write the problem in an unambiguous terms; he must define complex terminology, if any; he must formulate a clear-cut design and procedures for conducting research; he must present the tabulation of the result in an objective manner so also the summary and conclusion with scholarly caution.

Role of Statistics in Health Science Research

Statistical methodology finds its place wherever numerical facts enter into picture. Statistics is an integral part of biological research since it deals with various numerical aspects. Some of these are detailed below.

i. Research involves precise observation and accurate description as well as comparisons. This is possible only if information is collected in a scientifically designed pattern. Statistical methods help the research worker to suitably plan for the collection of desired information through appropriate statistical designs.

ii. Inherent feature of all biological observations is their variability. Each individual varies from one another with respect to different medical or biological phenomena. Similarly each group of individuals are different from other groups. As an example, the pulse rate, the haemoglobin level or the total number of white blood cells in a given volume of blood etc., vary from person to person even amongst healthy ones. Though a single fixed value for any of the above measurements cannot be called as a standard value for a healthy individual, a range can always be expressed as a standard or normal value. Again these ranges may vary from one group to the other due to various factors. As an example the pulse rate per minute of an individual varies from the infant age group to the older age group. Similarly the normal haemoglobin level varies from one part of the country to the other. As such in order to define these normal values and also to compare them from one group to another, Statistical Methodologies have an important application.

iii. Statistical quantities serve as indices for the measurement of health of a community in terms of rates and ratios of fatalities, morbidities, mortalities, health facilities and their availability or usage and so on. These indicators are useful in comparing the health status of a community or group from one place to the other or from one season or period to the other. They also help in analysing and interpreting the influence of environmental, social, economical, seasonal and other numerous factors on health of a community. As an illustration, prevalence of typhoid in a community may vary from one group of population to other. It may vary between different socio-economic groups or between seasons. The prevalence may also vary between those people who were not protected through immunisations as compared to those who were protected. By a systematic statistical analysis of the factors related to a disease, a health worker can define the problems in terms of such contrasts.

iv. Further there may be a number of factors responsible for the variations or contrasts in the health of a community. For example, the higher prevalence of typhoid amongst lower socio-economic group of the community may be due to lack of pure drinking water or consumption of unprotected food or lack of resistance due to under-nourishment or insufficient protection against disease because of non-acceptance of immunisation. By analysing the causes for such contrasts, with the help of Statistical Methodologies, effective control measures can be defined.

v. Statistical Methodologies are useful in the evaluation of health care delivery system or various preventive or control measures undertaken in a community, in an objective manner, since apparent changes in any of the factor may not be otherwise significant.

vi. Records of health care activities maintained and analysed statistically will help in understanding the health status of a community and also to assess the effectiveness of these programmes.

vii. Periodical investigations or surveys are undertaken in the community to define the problems and to elucidate the reasons for the contrasts. These investigations are planned and analysed using Statistical Methodologies.

viii. Statistical Methodologies play a vital role in planning and interpretation of epidemiological studies.
ix. Sophisticated Statistical Methodologies help in evolving suitable models for the delivery of health care activities.

Thus Statistical Methodologies are essential tools for planning of various research studies and interpretation of results of the studies.

2 Chapter
Types of Research

Research can be broadly of two types—*'Fundamental'* or *'Applied'*. When conducting fundamental research, the worker is investigating to obtain new knowledge on basic factors or principles governing the occurrence of various events. To quote an example, he may conduct a study to understand the changes in different physiological or biochemical responses in a particular disease condition as compared to normals. *Fundamental research* is a formal and systematic process. Here the researcher's aim is to develop a theory or a model by identifying all the important variables in a situation and discover broad generalisations and principles about the variables. It utilises a careful sample so that, conclusions can be generalised beyond the immediate situation. Fundamental research may not have concern with its immediate application.

In contrast to this type of research, it can be an *Applied research,* where the investigator applies the findings of the basic or fundamental research to understand the implications in real situations. This type of research tends to make generalisations about the populations and uses certain statistical techniques in selecting the sample for study. Here the main purpose is not to develop theories but to apply the theories to actual situations.

As an example, when it is known that a disease is caused because of a deficiency of a particular nutrient in food and if a research is undertaken to supplement this particular nutrient in the diseased persons, to understand the outcome of this procedure on the disease in relation to various other factors, the research is an applied one.

In health management, the research can be action oriented when it is known as *Action research.* In such a research the main emphasis would be to gain knowledge in undertaking different types of actions to increase the efficiency of the services. In Action research, researcher emphasises a problem which is immediate, urgent and has local application and focuses on the immediate consequences and applications of a problem and not on generalisations.

Research can also be *Operational research* where the investigator is investigating a particular set of actions to suggest improved efficiency in terms of certain defined parameters of outcome of such actions. Researcher focuses on finding out a best way of carrying out an activity when there are more than one option to attain a desired result when desired result is clearly defined. It involves a combination of research approaches. Operation research emphasises on taking decisions.

Depending on the nature of research, it can also be Experimental Research or Non-experimental Research. In Experimental Research, which may be either laboratory experiment or field experiment, independent variables can be manipulated where as in Non-experimental research independent variables cannot be manipulated. In Laboratory Research, experimenter can control the variables as needed and the results can be interpreted precisely under these conditions. Further experiments can be replicated to verify the result. Laboratory experiments have sufficient internal validity since extraneous variables can be controlled.

Field Experiments are carried out in realistic situations where independent variables cannot be manipulated. Common methods of field experiments are *descriptive studies* to describe certain phenomenon under realistic situations. They can also be *exploratory field studies* to understand the relationships amongst different variables so that a foundation is laid for formulating hypothesis, which may be further explored. Such studies only help to define the situations and relationship between variables but not to make any predictions.

Field experiments may be *hypothesis testing field studies,* where the researcher formulates certain hypothesis and collects evidence for testing the hypothesis. The advantages of such studies are that it provides an opportunity for direct observation of sociological interactions. They are carried out in realistic situations and continued observation in a given period of time is possible which provide a total picture of the social structure. However, due to complexity of precise measurement of all the variables, it may result in reducing internal validity. Further such studies may take long time and involve high cost.

These studies may be *Ex-post facto studies*, where the event has already occurred and only trace the events and no manipulation of variables are possible or may be *Prospective studies*, where the events are related to variables as they occur and there is possibility for manipulation of variables. These studies can be *Cross-sectional studies,* where the variables are studied as they are existing at the time of the study or *Longitudinal studies,* where the study is spread over a period of time and the outcome variables are studied as they occur or may be a *Cohort study,* where a specified group with *similar characteristics*, known as cohort is studied over a period of time and the outcome variables are studied as they occur.

Case studies are another type of research whose purpose is to understand aspects of the life cycle. This is one of the methods of non-experimental methods of research. In such research, certain cases or persons, families or communities are observed, and information is recorded using pre-designed questionnaires. Such studies are more descriptive.

Clinical trials are commonly used by clinicians. The main aim of a clinical trial is to make comparisons between one type of treatment with another. The parameters of these comparisons may be just in terms of certain physiological or biochemical estimates or may be in terms of number cured under different treatment groups. Such comparisons need careful thinking as well as scientific preplanning. A lot of variability exists within or between biological observations and this is even more predominant amongst clinical data. The effect of treatment for various diseases is not the same. As such the *Controlled clinical trials* play an important role in clinical experimentation.

Community health surveys are conducted to obtain a wide range of information on morbidity, mortality and other health conditions in the context of biological, social, environmental and economic factors and to bring to the surface priority problems of health care. Surveys are also conducted to evaluate the health measures undertaken. These health surveys can be broadly classified into three types. (i) general health surveys, (ii) comprehensive health surveys and (iii) morbidity surveys.

General health survey includes information on the components of health such as health status of the population including demographic indicators, morbidities, impairments, anthropometric data and mortalities, conditions influencing health especially the socio-economic conditions, nutrition, environmental factors, living habits and genetic factors, availability and utilisation of health services, health economics and evaluation of various health measures undertaken.

Comprehensive health survey is a multisubject or multipurpose or multistage survey to obtain information covered under general health survey. Besides information included in general health survey, additional information on other items such as constitutional provisions, training of medical and health personnel, availability of equipment and resources, health situation in the light of various health factors, existing medical and health facilities inclusive of inter-relationships and channels of communication are included.

Morbidity survey is a specific survey dealing with the collection of information on general morbidity or with a selected disease along with factors associated with the morbidity. When it is focussed on a selected disease or a problem it is called as special purpose survey.

Record analysis of the records maintained by agencies providing medical and health care is another method of research to obtain data about health status of a population. Medical and health records with hospitals, health centres, dispensaries, medical practitioners, social welfare agencies, records of births, deaths and records of notifiable diseases are examples of such records containing huge amount of useful information. Advantages of this method are that usually the quality of the diagnostic information is superior to that of interview method and the information obtained will be useful whenever the care provided by an institution is complete and if there are no other agencies from which the particular care is provided. However, the disadvantages of this method are that the population base, which is required for the calculation of various rates will not be available unless the institution completely covers a defined area. Further, all the desired information may not be available from the records as the records might not have been designed for the requirements of the survey.

Chapter 3 Planning of Research Studies

All research studies have to be designed in a systematic way to yield valid and reliable results. Unless these basic steps are followed, the research worker is bound to get into problems at the time of interpretation of results.

The basic steps involved in the formulation of a research protocol can be visualised as follows:

i. Definition of a problem for research
ii. Formulation of objectives and hypotheses
iii. Decision about the methodology of research for the particular problem
iv. Selection of variables for the study
v. Designing tools for data collection
vi. Definition of the study population, sample, controls, adequate sample size and time coverage
vii. Formulation of analytical methods of the data and planning for resources for analysis
viii. Anticipation of various possible errors and evolving appropriate actions to rectify the errors.

The detailed aspects of these steps are given below:

i. Definition of a Problem for Research

The basic step in the formulation of a research protocol is to define a suitable problem for the study. This is the most important and crucial part. In order to define the problem it is necessary to study the trends, patterns and changes, which have taken place in the subject of study. This will help to understand as to what has already been done, what has yet to be done and what are the priorities. A thorough knowledge on these aspects can be obtained through a detailed study of available literature and through discussions with peer groups.

Important sources for literature review are, different journals or periodicals pertaining to the area of research, reviews on the topic, books relating to the topic of research, various abstracts or indexes, research desertations or doctoral thesis.

While reviewing any scientific material, sufficient information should be recorded on the following items so that it would help in planning of a study. Problem investigated, objectives of study in brief, hypothesis formulated for the study, methodology adopted for the study, population and sample studied, nature of population, size of the sample, methods adopted for collection of data, manipulated and controlled variables, study designs and findings of the study relating to each hypothesis.

The problem for the study should be clearly specified in definite statements. There may be many unanswered areas in the field of study but the researcher has to direct his attention on a few of them at a time. Before defining the problem, it is opt to address questions such as, under which circumstances does a particular event seem to occur or what are the patterns related to such occurrence, etc. Before formulating the actual problem all related factors are to be clearly defined. Care should be taken to understand whether these factors are observable or measurable. While deciding about the problem, the feasibility in terms of resources like time, money, material and availability of subjects for study as well as methodologies for collection of data should also be kept in mind.

After careful study as above, one should clearly define the problem in specific and easily understandable words.

ii. Formulation of Objectives and Hypotheses

When a problem is selected and the factors, which are to be investigated, are identified, it is necessary to define the aims of study. In other words, it is necessary to define the details as to what the particular research is to achieve under each of the factors defined under the problem. This step will help the research worker to formulate the course of action to be taken under the research as well as to assess at the end, whether one has achieved what was desired. These objectives are to be defined in clear statements for each of the factors decided to be investigated. Such statements are known as hypothesis. Statement of hypothesis should be:

i. Simple and to the point
ii. Specific, not vague or general
iii. Conceptually clear i.e., properly expressed, with due care to use exact terms confirming to the existing concept
iv. Related to the available technique of measurement or experimentation or knowledge
v. Confirming to the body of existing theory and
vi. Capable of empirical test.

Ultimately, these hypotheses are going to be proved or disproved on the basis of the research investigation.

iii. Selection of Appropriate Methodologies of Research

The research protocol should take into consideration, the methodology of research to be followed. Various types of research, which can be undertaken, are already highlighted. The methodologies may vary according to the type of research. In clinical and paraclinical fields they may be mostly experimental under laboratory conditions while in preventive and health management they will be conducted under community settings.

iv. Selection of Variables for the Study

On the basis of defined objectives and hypotheses, one has to formulate a list of all relevant variables pertinent to the problem on which the data is to be collected. Only on the basis of these variables one has to decide about the tools as well as equipment for the collection of information. While deciding the variables it is necessary to keep in mind the feasibility of collecting the data in a reliable and accurate manner on the listed variables.

v. Designing Tools for Data Collection

After the variables are decided, the next step in the design of a research protocol is to equip oneself with all the tools, which are needed, for collecting information on the particular variables. Data for the study is collected either by laboratory experimentation or field studies. In a laboratory set up or clinical experimentation, they are the equipment while in survey methodologies they are the questionnaires or proforma for eliciting the data. Concepts influencing the variables are to be clearly defined and the techniques or methodologies of data collection are to be standardised. This will enable the researcher to maintain uniformity in results and will also help in getting measurements in a precise and accurate manner.

In the case of a survey, the questionnaire prepared should adhere to certain norms. The variables selected are to be arranged in a systematic way, preferably in a sequential order. In fact information on some of the variables may have to be collected through more than one question. Care has to be taken that the wordings of the question are non-ambiguous and non-controversial. The questions may be open ended where the answers to the questions are decided by the interviewee or they may be closed where the answers are predefined in terms of alternatives by the interviewer. Whenever, the questions are framed in terms of subjective answers, like satisfactory and unsatisfactory or mild, moderate and severe etc., definition of these terms are to be standardised to get uniform answers from all the interviewees.

When many variables are to be included in the study, care should be taken that the questionnaire does not become unduly long. In such cases the questionnaire has to be divided into more than one. The questionnaire is to be framed keeping in mind the facilities available for the analysis of data through manual tabulation or computer techniques.

Once the preliminary questionnaire is finalised it is to be pre-tested for its validity or reliability. In other words the questionnaire should provide data on what is actually desired in a manner that the same information is obtained on repeated administration of the questionnaire on the same population. This is possible by pretesting of the questionnaire through pilot studies and then suitably modifying the questionnaire on the basis of knowledge gained thereon.

vi. Selection of Population and Sample

Usually the study is undertaken on a group of animals or human beings, which are known as population for the study. The decision about the exact nature of the population has to be made on the basis of the problem and objectives of the study. The information obtained on a particular type of population may not be applicable to any other type. The main considerations which are to be kept in mind at the time of decision about the study population is the homogeneity with reference to independent variables. With human populations, care should be taken to select the appropriate groups like populations from the general community, hospital patients, institutional populations or special groups like factory workers, school children or population suffering from specified disease and so on. Population groups for the study may include certain *cohorts* where the population units will have common characteristics in terms of certain independent variables. Selection of the population groups for the study is done on the background of the objectives of the study.

Study can be conducted on the entire population if facilities are available which may not always exist. Otherwise samples are to be taken out of the entire population for the study. Such samples should be representative of the population. This will be possible if random samples are taken from the original populations. There are various random sampling designs which are appropriate under different circumstances which may be utilised for selecting suitable random samples. These methodologies are given in detail under the chapters on Sampling techniques and Design of Clinical Trials.

vii. Adequate Sample Size for the Study

Usual question to be answered while conducting an investigation is about the size of the sample or in other words, the number of units to be included in the sample. Bigger the sample size better will be the precision of the estimates from the sample. But due weight is to be given for the time, cost as well as practicability of investigating a big sample. Hence always an optimum size of the sample is to be considered keeping in view of the above factors.

The methodologies of estimation of adequate sample size are described under the chapters on Sampling Techniques and Design of Clinical Trials.

viii. Time Coverage for Data Collection

Time factor is an important consideration to be kept in mind especially for collection of data from the community studies. Most of the data follow either temporal trend over years or seasonal trend within a year.

As such the time scheduling for data collection has to be done in the light of objectives of the study. Further, one has to decide whether the study is going to be *cross sectional* i.e., pertaining to a specific point of time or is to be a *longitudinal* over a period of time. Cross sectional surveys are appropriate to estimate prevalence rates while longitudinal surveys are useful in estimating incidence rates or for studying patterns over a time period or for monitoring of different programmes.

ix. Other Factors to be Considered in Community Surveys

In the case of surveys, the design may be in terms of single or repeated visits to each household or person. It should also be decided whether the questions are to be asked as listed in the questionnaire or some sort of probe questions or structured questions will be put to the interviewee. The selection of the respondent who is to be interviewed is also very important. The respondent's level of knowledge of the events, memory of events and responsibility in giving the correct information should be kept in mind while selecting the respondent. The recall period for various items should not be too long otherwise the chances of under estimation due to memory factor will be very high. The selection and training of technical staff, the quantity of work to be assigned to them, the quality control methods for the collected data, an advance idea about tabulation and analysis procedures are some of the other factors, which are to be kept in mind at the stage of planning of the investigations. If the analysis procedures are not comprehended at the time of planning of a research study, one may end up with a situation that suitable data may not be available for the desired analysis.

x. Controlling Errors in the Study

Usually two types of errors can occur in the course of an investigation. First type of error is the response error which will come up if the sample is not completely covered due to either non cooperation or mortality of experimental units during the course of investigation. This error can be reduced by perseverant efforts of the investigator to reduce the non co-operation or by proper planning of the sample size allowing for such non-responses due to mortality, etc. The quantum of this error can also be estimated by conducting a repeat study on non-respondents and applying suitable corrections for the estimates from the results of the repeat study. The second type of error may be due to faulty techniques and or errors in measurement and recording. These can be reduced by standardisation of techniques and proper training of personnel.

4 Chapter — Collection of Data

Types of Data

Before going into the actual details of collection of data, it is necessary to understand the meaning of data and various types of data. Whenever an observation is made, it will be recorded and a collective recording of these observations either numerical or otherwise is called as Data. These observations may be collected in a simple way like recording the sex of a person in a group or noting down the number of cases of a disease in a community or may be done through an experiment such as counting the total white blood cells in a given volume of blood, etc. of an individual. In each of the above cases a certain observation is made of a characteristic and this characteristic which varies from one observation to the other is called as a *variable.*

Depending upon the nature of the variable, the data is classified as *Qualitative* or *Quantitative*. When the data is recorded in a qualitative form like sex, type of disease, cause of death, etc. the data is termed as Qualitative Data. When the variable under observation takes quantitative values like haemoglobin level or white blood cell count in a given volume of blood, etc. the data is called as Quantitative Data. Ordinarily in a qualitative data the observations are obtained by enumeration or counting while in a quantitative data the observations are obtained through certain measurements.

Quantitative data can be further classified into two kinds, namely *discrete* and *continuous*. When the variable under observation can take only fixed values in a given range like whole numbers or the variable jumps from one number to another without taking in between values, the data is called as *Discrete data*. Instead, if the variable can take any value in the given range of numbers, the data is called as *Continuous data*. As specific examples, the number of white blood cells in a given volume of blood is a discrete data as it can be expressed only in whole numbers while the haemoglobin percentage level of an individual is a continuous data as it can be measured to any decimal value depending on the precision of the measuring instruments.

In Health sciences, data may be collected either for research or for defining health status of a population or for monitoring of health activities. In all these, the data is obtained from various sources by actual experimentation or through surveys or analysis of records.

Methods of Data Collection for Field Studies

i. Concepts of Data Collection

The data for any research study can be collected either from primary source known as *Primary data or* secondary source known as *Secondary data*. Primary data are those which are collected afresh or for the first time while Secondary data are those, which are collected from data already available from other sources such as institutional records, published reports or studies.

Data can be collected either by *Quantitative* or by *Qualitative* method. Quantitative methods are adopted to obtain information of descriptive type and will provide data for estimations. These may be either Survey method or Experimentation. Qualitative methods of data collection are for understanding underlying causes of occurrence of a phenomenon or a particular event. It will provide information to understand *"WHY"* of an event. The method seeks to understand the behavioural patterns such as beliefs, actions or norms of subjects under study. Usually the method does not provide data for making estimations.

Quantitative methods of data collection should confirm to the following principles:

a. Sample should be representative and preferably of large size.

b. Should adopt standardised individual questionnaires.
c. Only limited number of variables of interest are studied.
d. Information collected should be quantifiable and amenable to statistical procedures.

In contrast to above principles, in qualitative methods of data collection :

a. Sample is purposive.
b. Methods adopted are interviews, either of individuals or groups, observations, case studies or group discussions.
c. Information obtained is extensive, descriptive and subjective, but may not be amenable to routine statistical analytical methods.
d. Relationship with the respondent is structured or semi-structured.
e. Method tries to get the inside of the interviewee's world.

ii. Quantitative Methods of Data Collection

Important methods of collection of quantitative data are:

a. Interview method
b. Observation method
c. Questionnaire method

Selection of appropriate method depends on nature and scope of the study, availability of funds, availability of time and precision of estimates to be made from the data.

a. Interview Method

Interview method is the most commonly used method in field studies. It involves presentation of oral-verbal stimuli and reply in terms of oral-verbal responses. The interviews may be personal interviews or telephonic interviews. Personal interviews are usually carried out in a structured way and are known as *Structured interviews.* In this technique predetermined questions are asked and recorded on a pre-designed and pre-tested proforma. *Unstructured interviews* do not follow a system of predetermined order of questioning. However, unstructured interviews require deep knowledge on the subject.

The advantages of interview method of data collection are:

i.More information in greater depth can be obtained.

ii. Interviewer with his skill can overcome the resistance from the respondent.
iii. Has greater flexibility and questions can be restructured as per situations.
iv. Personal information can be obtained.
v. Samples can be covered completely with repeated visits.
vi. Interviewer can capture lot of information.
vii. Can also collect supplementary information.
viii. Desired information can be collected at one point.
ix. Provides accurate data for calculation of various rates or ratios.

However the method is expensive and time consuming. Great care has to be taken to avoid interviewer's bias as well as interviewee's bias. This can be attained by careful selection and training of interviewers. The method involves establishment of good rapport with the interviewee.

b. Observation Method

This is a common method used in behavioural sciences or clinical case studies where information is obtained by investigator's own observation. Before starting observation it is necessary to make a checklist of items to be observed as well as structuring the style of recording to facilitate easy analysis.

The advantages of this method are that subjective bias of both observer and respondent is eliminated since information pertains to what is happening. Further the observations are independent of respondents willingness to answer questions. This method is useful especially when the respondents are not capable of answering verbal question.

However the method is expensive, information provided is limited and sometimes unforeseen factors may interfere with observation. In some cases respondents may not be willing to be observed.

The observation may be *Participant observation* where the observer shares the experiences, being a member of the group. It may be a *Non participant observation* when the observer is a detached emissary. It may also be *Disguised observation* when the observations are made without people knowing that they are being observed.

c. Questionnaire Method

In this method a pre-designed and pre-tested questionnaire is circulated to the respondents, either in person or through mail, who will answer the questions by themselves. The answers to the questions may be structured or open ended. This method is less expensive compared to other methods since questionnaires can be circulated to large samples. However the method has the disadvantage of loss of coverage since all the respondents may not return the questionnaires. Further all the questions may not be answered by all the respondents. Besides, there may be difficulty in understanding the questions by the respondents. This can be taken care of by adopting *guided questionnaire* method where the group of respondents are initially briefed about the questions.

iii. Qualitative Methods of Data Collection

Commonly used qualitative methods are:
a. Case study method
b. Focus group discussions

a. Case Study Method

This is a popular form of qualitative method of data collection and is a systematic research technique used extensively by sociologists, behavioural scientists and anthropologists and even clinicians. The method involves complete and careful observation of a community, social unit, institution, family, individual or an episode or an event in the life of an individual. Usually an in-depth analysis of a limited number of variables and their interrelationships are carried out. The method is more for understanding the behaviour patterns, cause and effect and to formulate hypothesis, which can be tested through a detailed study to generalise the observations.

Major Advantages of case study technique are that, it helps to understand the behavioural patterns, collect personal data, trace the natural history of the event and their relationship with other factors, study intensively the social units and to provide a basis for formulation of further studies.

However through case studies it may not be possible to arrive at generalisations since the data pertains only to the case under study which may not be a representative sample.

b. Focus Group Discussions

The method is a semistructured discussion of a given topic with a homogeneous group of 6 to 10 individuals. In this method the discussions are not rigidly controlled as in the case of an interview using a standardised questionnaire, but is neither an unstructured conversation. The discussion is led by a trained *facilitator* who uses a checklist of items to be discussed and encourages the participants to respond to open ended questions and to come out with their responses.

Advantages of focus group discussions are that the group members can spontaneously express their ideas and they are not pressurised to answer questions. The flexible format allows the facilitator to explore the situations in an open manner. A wide range of information can be elicited in a less expensive manner.

However, the limitations of group discussions are that the information elicited may not be representative of the population and special statistical techniques are to be used for analysis. The analysis and interpretation of information elicited is more subjective.

Various steps and tasks involved in any focus group discussions are as follows—

i. Definition of the topic for discussions and identifying information to be collected

Broad topic should be determined based upon priorities. In a single study it is not possible to collect vast information in in-depth manner. As such a choice has to be made between range of topics and the depth of information to be collected within the limited time.

ii. Constitution of study team

The constitution of the study team should be based on the skills of the team members in planning and conducting group discussions. The team should have sufficient understanding of the content and priorities of information to be collected, skills in qualitative data collection methods, familiarity with the communities or target groups to be interviewed, fluency in local language and organisational capabilities.

iii. Development of a scheme for information collection

Development of a scheme of information collection will enable the team to visualise the scope of the information to be collected as well as help them to think holistically about different aspects of the subject matter to be studied, as the focus group discussions are aimed at discovering different aspects of the situations. This scheme should include main items and sub items to be covered in a systematic manner. While formulating these details interrelationship of information to be collected should be kept in mind. It is better to visualise the scheme in a flow chart format indicating the sequencing of information to be collected.

iv. Identifying target groups and sample of interviewees

Identification of targets groups who are to be included in the group is very crucial. This should be influenced by the fact on the knowledge of the group about the desired information covered under the topic for investigation. In deciding about the target groups, practical considerations of time and resource should also be kept in mind. Thus data collection should concentrate on those groups who are most knowledgeable as well as influential on the topic of investigation. The number of groups to be interviewed should be a minimum of three groups of each type. The sample size for any group interview should be limited to 6 to 10 persons per group. The basic principle to decide on the composition of a group is homogeneity of group members. People will feel more comfortable and respond freely in groups who are similar with respect to age, sex, socio-economic status, etc.

v. Formulation of group interview guide and questions

The interview guide should be in terms of series of questions to be covered during the discussions. This guide should be flexible and adoptive as per situations. Questions formulated should be in third person, usually hypothetical, and explore basic aspirations and anxieties. The questions should be in the local language and dialect of the respondents. Most of the questions should be open ended and should not lead to definite conclusions. The questions are to be clearly worded in an understandable manner, neutral so that it would not influence the answer, formulated in a positive rather than in a negative manner. The questions are to be sequenced in an answerable manner.

vi. Notes taking during interviews

The notes should be taken during interviews in as detailed manner as possible. The notes should reflect exactly as to what the participants say *verbatim* and should not be filtered. Notes should be taken in first person, key words and ideas should be recorded, original sayings and phrasings should be retained, should be worded exactly as spoken and should reflect different opinions expressed by the group.

vii. Other aspects of conducting a group interview

The spot selected for interview should not be controversial and should be neutral facilitating all the participants to gather, besides being less disturbing and distracting.

Participants should sit in a circle, facing each other, so that proper interaction is ensured between the participants.

The facilitator should sit in the same level as the other participants to identify himself as one of them.

It is important to greet the participants, explain them the purpose of the interview and assure them that the responses would be kept anonymous.

Interviews should be limited to a maximum of about one to one and half hours.

Tools Preparation for Data Collection

Tools may be questionnaires or schedules or proforma for field investigations, through which the desired information is collected and recorded. They contain the variables in question form. The answers to the questions are recorded in either a pre-structured or unstructured form. Pre-structured refers to the answers in a pre-designed form while unstructured means open ended answers. Tools developed should have *validity* and *reliability.* Validity refers to the collection of desired information in complete and true form, while reliability refers to obtaining same answers, when information is collected again for a particular question from the same respondent. While designing tools the following aspects are to be kept under consideration:

i. Objectives of the study are to be clearly stated.
ii. Tools should be prepared keeping in mind type of respondents, nature of information and method of analysis to be adopted.
iii. All the variables to be covered under the study are to be listed in advance.
iv. Questions pertaining to the listed variables are framed in a simple and understandable form and are to be logically sequenced. Sometimes particular variable may require more than one question.
v. The tools designed are to be pre-tested through *Pilot studies* for testing for validity and reliability. Pre-testing will also help the investigator to understand other aspects such as time required for each interview and other practical aspects.
vi. Tools are to be thoroughly edited on the basis of results of pre-testing.
vii. Questionnaires should not be lengthy and they are to be split into more number of simple ones.
viii. Questions are to be well framed in an understandable manner and should be simple and straight forward.
ix. Subjective questions should have clear cut definitions for their classifications to attain uniformity in answers.
x. In structured tools, the pre-designed answers should be

clearly defined to avoid subjectivity and to enable collection of information in a uniform pattern.

xi. It would be advantageous for analysis, if computerised format is used for data collection.

Collection of Morbidity Data

There is no regular system for the collection of morbidity data either at state or national level. Still major health institutions compile the outpatient and in patient records according to the names of the diseases. From these reports the Central Bureau of Health Intelligence attached to the Director General of Health Services publishes periodical reports after compiling and collating health data from various sources.

Periodical or ad-hoc surveys are also undertaken by organisations like Central Statistical Organisation, National Sample Survey Wing of Cabinet Secretariat, Indian Council of Medical Research, etc. to obtain information on various morbidities.

Further information regarding communicable diseases is compiled from the reports of infectious diseases.

Morbidity information can also be obtained from :

i. Hospital and dispensary records
ii. General practitioners records
iii. Records of health and welfare centres and educational institutions
iv. Recruitment and sickness records of Armed forces
v. Records of social security schemes such as Employees State insurance scheme, Contributory health service scheme, Life insurance, etc.
vi. Records of notifiable diseases
vii. Reports of routine and special sickness surveys
viii. Statistical abstracts of important diseases
ix. Statistical reports of important health institutions
x. Reports of registries established for certain diseases like cancer.

Chapter 5

Tabulation of Data

Raw data as recorded in a proforma will not be of much help in understanding their meaning or underlying trends. As such the data should be arranged and classified in a suitable manner. A preliminary and convenient way of presentation of data is to arrange them in the form of tables. Data can be arranged into different types of tables depending upon the nature of data and purpose of tabulation.

Frequency Distribution Table

In a frequency distribution (Table 5.1), the observations are arranged into a table depicting the value of the variable according to number of times the particular value has occurred in the series, as depicted below.

Table 5.1: Frequency distribution of individuals in a community according to the number of illness suffered by them in a year

No. of illness suffered in a year	No. of individuals	
	No.	Per cent
0	24	4.7
1	76	14.9
2	114	22.4
3	115	22.5
4	86	16.9
5	51	10.0
6	26	5.1
7	18	3.5
Total	**510**	**100.0**

In Table 5.1, the data of the number of illness suffered by individual members has been arranged into a table. When the raw data of 510 members is viewed individually, it will not mean anything. But after arranging the data into the above table it can be easily understood that only 24 or 4.7% of members did not have any illness, 76 or 14.9% had one illness, 114 or 22.4% had two illnesses and that almost same number, had three illnesses. From the Table 5.1 it can also be inferred that maximum number of members had two to four illnesses and the number of illnesses extends up to 6 or 7 in a year.

The above table is the most common way of presentation of data in the form of tables and is known as *frequency distribution* table. It can be seen from the table that the first column consists of values of the variable and adjoining column consists of the number of times the particular value of variable has occurred or in other words the frequency of occurrence of the value of the variable in the series of data.

Above data is discrete data and also the values of variable have a small range. If on the other hand, the variable is continuous or has a large range, the table, if presented in terms of single values of the variable, the table becomes very long and will not help in making inferences from the table. For such data the table is prepared after grouping the values of variable. Such groups are known as *class-intervals.*

Table 5.2: Frequency distribution of haemoglobin level of antenatal mothers in a community

Hb. level in gm%	No. of mothers	
	No.	Per cent
8.1 - 9.0	13	6.0
9.1 - 10.0	20	9.3
10.1 - 11.0	25	11.6
11.1 - 12.0	35	16.2
12.1 - 13.0	48	22.2
13.1 - 14.0	35	16.2
14.1 - 15.0	22	10.2
15.1 - 16.0	18	8.3
Total	**216**	**100.0**

In Table 5.2, frequency distribution of haemoglobin level of antenatal mothers is presented. Since the haemoglobin level is measured in decimals one gm% is taken as a class interval. From the table, it can be inferred that majority of mothers, that is, 54.6% are in the haemoglobin range 11.1 to 14.0 gms%, while 15.3% are up to only 10.0 gm%. Thus the table helps in understanding the patterns quickly.

Multiple Classification

When two or more variables are under study, the variables can be simultaneously presented in the same table. The variables are classified both along the rows and columns and the frequency corresponding to each pair of values of the variables is presented in a cell. An illustration of a two-way classification is presented in Table 5.3.

Table 5.3: Distribution of height and weight of students aged seventeen years in a class

Height in cm Weight in kg	41-45	46-50	51-55	56-60	61-65	66-70	Total
146-150	—	—	1	—	—	—	1
151-155	2	1	1	—	1	—	5
156-160	8	12	11	2	2	2	37
161-165	7	23	40	15	5	—	90
166-170	2	8	18	14	6	1	49
171-175	1	1	8	10	5	3	28
Total	**20**	**45**	**79**	**41**	**19**	**6**	**210**

This table presents the data on height and weight of students in a class. Each cell gives the number of students corresponding to the height and weight of the particular row and column.

For example the cell corresponding to the third row and first column, indicates that there are eight students corresponding to a weight of 41-45 kg. and height of 156-160 cm. Similarly, observations can be made for any cell corresponding to the weight and height of that cell. The last row and the last column, known as marginal totals, give the frequency distribution of height and weight of students respectively.

It may be observed that the data presented in the above tables are quantitative in nature. Qualitative data can also be presented in similar tables. As an example the blood group distribution of individuals without leprosy and different types of leprosy (Table 5.4) is presented to understand whether there is any association between blood group and incidence of leprosy in individuals.

Table 5.4: Distribution of blood groups amongst a sample of persons without leprosy and patients with different types of leprosy

Blood Group	Individuals classified as						
	Without leprosy		Lepromatous leprosy		Non-lepromatous leprosy		Total
	No.	Percent	No.	Percent	No.	Percent	
A	30	20.0	49	29.0	52	34.2	131
B	60	40.0	49	29.0	36	23.7	145
O	47	31.3	59	34.9	48	31.6	154
AB	13	8.7	12	7.1	16	10.5	41
Total	**150**	**100.0**	**169**	**100.0**	**152**	**100.0**	**471**

From the above table, a preliminary observation can be made that the distribution pattern of blood group is not same with persons without leprosy and leprosy patients. Further it suggests that the proportion of persons with 'A' blood group are more amongst leprosy patients as compared to persons without leprosy, while 'B' blood group is more common amongst persons without leprosy as compared to patients with leprosy .

Tables can also be prepared for summary statistics of observations as tabulated in Table 5.5. In the table, summary parameters, Mean and Standard Deviation (SD) of certain assessment parameters at different intervals of time in a study relating to effect of anti-hypertensive drugs is presented.

Table 5.5: Statistical parameters of assessment at different intervals

Parameters of assessment	At start		After 6 hours		After 12 hours	
	Mean	SD	Mean	S D	Mean	S D
Systolic BP	192	19.1	170	18.8	140	18.9
Diastolic BP	120	8.3	117	7.5	100	7.2
Heart rate	87	10.2	88	18.6	81	8.3

Basic Principles of Tabulation of Data

i. Every table should contain a title indicating as what has been presented in the table. Ordinarily, titles should be brief and to the point. Title can be written either at the top or bottom.
ii. The number of class intervals in a table should not be too many or too less. Depending on the aims of presentation, the number of class intervals may be decided. Class intervals may be equal or unequal depending on the purpose of presentation.
iii. Rows and columns are to be clearly defined as to what is presented in them.
iv. Standard codes and symbols are to be used and wherever necessary, they are to be explained as footnotes.
v. Units of measurement of variables are to be specified.
vi. The end and beginning points of class intervals should not be overlapping.
vii. If the data presented is of secondary sources, the source of data should be mentioned at the bottom of the table.

The above hints, aim at making the table self-explanatory.

Working Method for Tabulation of Data

The data available on proforma, schedules or registers are transformed into tables mainly by two methods. One is known as *manual tabulation* using tally marks method and the other through computers. The manual tabulation method is appropriate when the volume of data, both in terms of number of variables as well as number of observations, is not large. Otherwise computers are used to generate tables. Statistical packages are available for the purpose. When computers are used, the data is to be transferred on to computers in specified pattern according to the Statistical package used for analysis.

Manual or Tally Marks Method of Tabulation

First the range for the values of the variable is noted. Then this range is divided into suitable number of groups so that the number of groups is neither many nor less to enable suitable conclusions. These groups or class intervals are noted down in the first column of the table. Then each observation is tabulated into these class intervals, in the second column by a tally mark. This is done by going through the data in a sequential manner and putting a tally against the class interval corresponding to the value of the variable. A fifth tally is put for every fifth observation in the class interval across the previous four tallies to enable easy counting of tallies.

One has to be careful in putting tallies, and if a mistake is committed, entire process has to be repeated.

Tabulation by the above procedure is illustrated for the data in Example 5.1.

Example 5.1. WBC count per cu. mm. of blood for a group of individuals are as follows—

6200	5400	8000	7000	6000	5650	6550	7540
4250	6270	7570	7250	4675	5750	6500	4800
4020	6580	7950	6550	8200	6500	8500	6500
6500	8500	7200	5000	7000	5500	7400	7500
5500	8250	5190	8450	8000	6250	7550	6800
7600	6500	8500	8500	8300	8200	6500	6600
6500	4600	4800	5200	6650	7500	6800	5800
7500	8000	8500	7750	6750	5850	7400	4900
5200	6750	5850	6250	5850	5750	5600	4800
7350	7540	6540	6970	7460	4560	7900	7500

Nine class intervals as given in column of Table 5.6. can be formed. These class intervals are written in the first column. Then the data is read one by one, may be in terms of rows. The first observation is 6200 and a tally mark is put against the class interval 6001-6500. The second observation is 5400 and a tally is marked against the class interval 5001-5500. The third is 8000 for which tally is marked against the class interval 7501-8000. Thus the procedure is repeated for all observations. When all the tallies are marked for the data the table will be as shown in Table 5.6.

Table 5.6: Preliminary table for the WBC count of a group of individuals

WBC count per cu. mm. of blood	Tally marks	Frequency
4001-4500	//	2
4501-5000	~~////~~ ///	8
5001-5500	~~////~~ /	6
5501-6000	~~////~~ ////	9
6001-6500	~~////~~ ~~////~~ /	11
6501-7000	~~////~~ ~~////~~ ///	13
7001-7500	~~////~~ ~~////~~ /	11
7501-8000	~~////~~ ~~////~~	10
8001-8500	~~////~~ ~~////~~	10
Total		**80**

Then a final table is prepared as detailed earlier.

Classification of Diseases, Injuries and Causes of Death, Age and Occupation

While tabulating data on morbidities, mortalities, age, occupation, etc. a standard classification has to be followed so as to enable comparisons from one research study to other. International organisations like World Health Organisation, International Labour Organisation and National Organisations like Census Directorate have adopted certain standard classifications, which are given below :

i. Classification of Diseases, Injuries and Causes of Deaths

World Health Organisation has recommended classifications for the above data. They are revised once in ten years. Presently tenth revision is in use.

The structure of the tenth revision retains the basic classification originally proposed by William Farr in the early days of disease classification. His scheme of classification was based on grouping the diseases as epidemic diseases, constitutional or general diseases, local diseases arranged by site, developmental diseases and injuries. The classification system adopted is basically a single coded list of three character categories, each of which can be further divided into up to ten four character subcategories. Tenth revision uses an alphanumeric code with a letter in the first position and a number in the second, third and fourth positions. The fourth character follows a decimal point. Possible codes range from A00.0 to Z99.9.

WHO has published these classifications in three volumes.

Tabular lists of WHO is contained in Volume 1 providing main classification composed of the list of three character categories and the tabular list of inclusions and four character subcategories.

Volume 3 contains an alphabetical index of all diseases.

WHO classification has twenty one main categories as follows—

I Certain infections and parasitic diseases
II Neoplasms
III Diseases of the blood and blood forming organs and certain disorders involving the immune mechanism
IV Endocrine, nutritional and metabolic diseases
V Mental and behavioural disorders
VI Diseases of nervous system
VII Diseases of the eye and adnexia
VIII Diseases of the ear and mastoid process
IX Diseases of the circulatory system
X Diseases of respiratory system
XI Diseases of digestive system
XII Diseases of skin and subcutaneous tissue
XIII Diseases of musculoskeletal system and connective tissue
XIV Diseases of genitourinary system
XV Pregnancy, child birth and the puerperium
XVI Certain conditions originating in the perinatal period
XVII Congenital malformations, deformations and chromosomal abnormalities
XVIII Symptoms, signs and abnormal clinical and laboratory findings, not elsewhere classified
XIX Injury and poisoning and certain other consequences of external causes
XX External causes of morbidity and mortality
XXI Factors influencing health status and contact with health services.

For detailed reporting of morbidity, tabulation lists are provided with 298 detailed items. There are lists for routine reporting as well as special tabulation lists, providing information on the most important diseases and external causes of death.

ii. Age Classification

Age statistics are important since most of the socio-demographic, morbidity and mortality analysis is performed according to age and sex variables. Information on age is highly deceptive and care is to be taken to elicit correct age. Always age at last birth day, i.e. the age in completed years, should be collected, except for infants, where it will be in completed months. There is a tendency in illiterates to give the age in years ending with 5 years. To take this error into consideration age classifications are mostly done in five year groups.

Classification of data on age is done keeping in mind the purpose and utility of the tabulation. The age classification should facilitate comparison of one set of data with the other. As such WHO has recommended classification as follows—

(a) For general purposes

- Under 1 year, single years to four years inclusive, five year groups from 5 to 84 years, 85 years and over.
- Under 1 year, 1 to 4 years, 5 to 14 years, 15 to 24 years, 25 to 34 years, 35 to 44 years, 45 to 54 years, 55 to 64 years, 65 to 74 years , 75 years and over.
- Under 1 year, 1 to 14 years, 15 to 44 years, 45 to 64 years, 65 years and over.

(b) For special statistics of infant mortality

- By single days for the first week of life, 7 to 13 days, 14 to 20 days, 21 to 27 days, 28 days up to but not including 2 months, by single months of life from 2 months to 1 year.
- Under 24 hours, 1 to 6 days, 7 to 21 days, 28 days up to but not including 3 months, 3 to 5 months, 6 months and over but under 1 year.
- Under 7 days, 7 to 27 days, 28 days upto but under 1 year.

If the age groups are tabulated in greater detail than in one of the above groupings specified above, they shall be arranged as to allow condensation into one of the above groups.

iii. Classification of Occupations

The International Labour Organisation (ILO) and the Director of Census Operations in India have provided classification lists for occupations. The list provided by ILO consists of ten major groups and each is further subdivided into two digit classification. The Indian census reports follow the same classification. The ten major classifications of workers and non workers are as follows—

i. Cultivators
ii. Agricultural labourers
iii. Livestock, Fishing, Plantations, etc
iv. Mining and Quarrying
v. Manufacturing, Processing, Servicing and Repairs
vi. Construction
vii. Trade and Commerce
viii. Transport, Storage and Communication
ix. Other Services
x. Non workers.

6 Chapter
Graphical Presentation of Data

Basic Concepts in Graphical Presentation

It is seen that the simplest method by which an unwieldy and complex data can be made understandable is by arranging the data into a suitable table. But it is also known that in tables there will be certain number of rows and columns and as such most of the times, it will be difficult to understand and visualise the comparisons and contrasts between two or more tables. It is always easier to grasp the data through visual inspection by suitable diagrams or graphs drawn for the data. As such diagrams are more useful methods of rendering the whole data readily intelligible to the eye. At the same time, because of their visual appeal, great care should be taken in designing the graphs so that the reader is not misled. As every aspect of the data cannot be presented in the diagrams, the graphs or diagrams will serve only as a preliminary aid in understanding of the data and to compare different sets of data. In the words of R.A. Fisher, "Diagrams prove nothing but they bring outstanding features to the eye. They are therefore no substitute for critical tests that may be applied to the data, but they are valuable in suggesting such tests explaining conclusions founded upon them."

The following are some of the important points to be remembered in the construction of diagrams and graphs.

i. The diagram should be simple and consistent with the type of data.
ii. Diagrams should be self-explanatory and should contain a brief and clear title of caption, the nature of the data, the coverage of data illustrating to what or to whom the

data relate, the period to which the data relate, the scale, index, etc.

iii. The number of lines drawn in any one graph should not be many so that the diagram does not look clumsy and should facilitate easy grasp of the salient features of the data.

iv. Usually the rulings of the graph paper should be light and the lines of the diagram should be heavier.

v. Ordinarily the values of the variables are represented on the horizontal or X-axis and the corresponding frequencies on the vertical or Y-axis.

vi. On both X-axis and Y-axis the scale of division of axis should be proportional and the division should be marked along with the details of the variable and frequencies, which are presented on the axis.

vii. Every graph should contain a brief title at the top and the scale of division for X-axis and Y-axis should be given at the right hand corner of graph.

viii. The lines drawn on a graph should never be extrapolated beyond the range of the values of the variable for which the graph is drawn.

Types of Diagrams

i. Line Diagram

This is the simplest type of diagram and is useful to study the changes of values of the variable with the passage of time. This diagram is drawn by presenting the time, such as hours, days, weeks, months, or years along the horizontal axis and the value of any quantity or index pertaining to this period along the vertical axis. The height or distance of each point from the base is represented by the value of the quantity studied at that particular point of time. When all such points corresponding to the time periods are plotted, they are joined by a line.

In this type of graph, the attention is towards the height of the curve at various points of the base or in other words towards the trend of the line drawn with the passage of time.

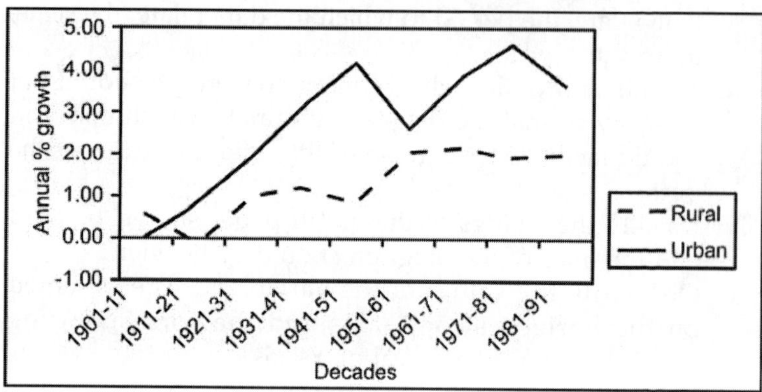

Fig. 6.1: Decadal growth of Indian population during 1901 to 1991

If more than one set of observations are to be compared on the same graph paper, then each set of observations is represented by a different type of line such as dotted line for one set of observations, broken line for another set and so on.

In Figure 6.1, the data pertaining to annual growth rates of India for urban and rural areas during different decades are presented. This graph shows the trend of these rates with the passage of time. This type of graph is useful to know the trend of the values of the variable over time. From the graph it can be seen that the urban areas are growing at a faster rate than rural areas. For rural areas, there was decline in these rates during 1911-21 and 1941-51, with a negative rate during 1911-21 while urban areas showed a decline only in 1951-61 and 1981-91.

ii. Logarithmic Scale for Line Diagram

In some cases instead of knowing the trend of variation of a particular variable over a period of time, it may be required to study the rate of change of the variable with the change in the time.

This rate of change may be of two types. In one case the variable may change with a constant addition for every unit of change in the other variable. In such cases, they are said to change in *arithmetic progression*. As an example the height of a person, up to a certain age, may increase in constant addition for every additional unit of age, say years. That is to say that the height at any age will be the height at the previous year plus the constant addition of height per year of age. When such data is plotted on ordinary graph paper, the diagram will be a straight line.

On the other hand, in certain types of observations, the change in one variable may occur as a constant multiple of the value of the variable at the previous point. In such cases the variable is said to be in *geometric progression*. As an example while measuring the toxicity of a drug on animals, it may happen that the number of animals, which die at a particular concentration of the drug, may be in certain multiple of the number of animals, which have died at the previous concentration of the drug. When such data is plotted on an ordinary graph paper the diagram will not be a straight line. In order to know the rate of change of the dependent variable in terms of the independent variable, from the graph, these graphs should be in the form of straight lines.

The rate of change can be measured from the angle between the straight line and the X-axis. To adjust for such data, usually the scale of one of the axes will be in ordinary scale while that of the other axis will be in logarithmic scale. Such graph papers are known as semi-log graph papers or *arith-log graph* papers.

Example of the application of such graphs in medicine is the log-dose response curves in Pharmacology. If the response to several doses of a particular drug is plotted against the doses, usually the graph will not be a straight line. But on the other hand, if log doses are taken and the corresponding responses are plotted then the graph obtained will be a straight line instead of taking logarithms of dose, the doses can be directly plotted on arith-log graph paper.

Here the doses are plotted on logarithmic scale axis while the response is plotted on arithmetic scale axis. Survival rates of organism for two treatments over a period of time depicted in Figure 6.2 on logarithmic scale, facilitates conclusions on the efficacy of drugs.

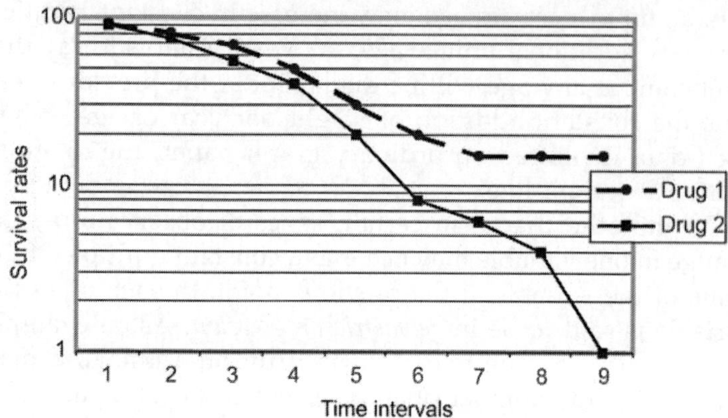

Fig. 6.2: Survival rate of organisms for two drugs at different three hourly intervals of time

iii. Bar Diagram

This graph is drawn from the frequency distribution table representing the variable on the horizontal axis and the frequency on the vertical axis. Bars or rectangles are drawn along the graph sheet. Height of each bar or rectangle corresponds to the frequency in a class interval in the case of quantitative data. In the case of qualitative data it corresponds to the frequency in each group of the characteristic under observation. The height of the rectangle of the bar will be corresponding to the frequency while the breadth or the base corresponds to the length of the class interval of the variable, if the graph is for quantitative data. In the case of qualitative data the breadth corresponds to the various groups or characteristics.

An illustration of this graph is shown in Figure 6.3 where the pattern of health care utilisation for sickness episodes in Karnataka State as revealed in a household health utilisation survey during a period is depicted.

The principle behind drawing the rectangles in this graph is that the height of the rectangle will be in proportion to the corresponding frequencies of the variable. The width of the base of all the rectangles drawn on a particular graph paper should be same when they are drawn for qualitative data.

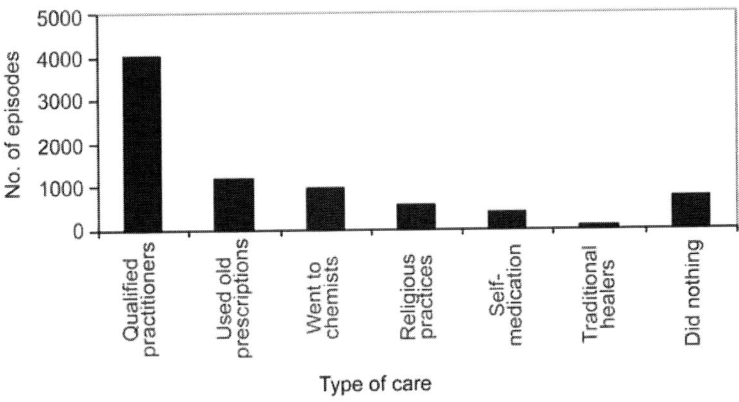

Fig. 6.3: Health care utilisation pattern for sickness episodes in Karnataka state during a period

In quantitative data they correspond to the width of the class interval as already stated. The different bars should normally be separated by equal spacing.

By comparing the height of the rectangles, comparisons of different groups can be made. As already seen, this graph can be used to depict qualitative data as well as quantitative data of discrete type.

Study of sub classification of qualitative data can be done by drawing separate bars corresponding to each subcategory. Separate shades are given for each bar. There will be as many shades as there will be sub portions in a group of data. Each of the shade should be indexed separately to make the graph easily understandable. Figure 6.4 is an example of depicting *Multiple bar diagram* of pattern of health care utilisation for sickness episodes in different divisions of Karnataka State as revealed in a household health utilisation survey.

iv. Proportional Bar Diagram

When it is desired to compare the proportion of frequencies within subgroups between different major groups of observations then bars are drawn for each major group with equal height and these bars are divided corresponding to subgroup proportions in each of major group. Each bar

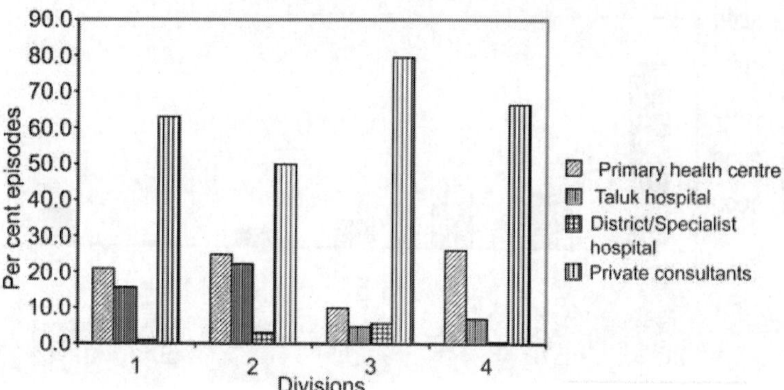

Fig. 6.4: Multiple bar diagram for the place of treatment for OPD consultations in different divisions of Karnataka

represents 100 per cent as their height. Within each bar various subgroups represents percentage of the frequencies in that particular subgroup.

In Figure 6.5 the Proportional bar diagram is drawn for the data of Figure 6.4.

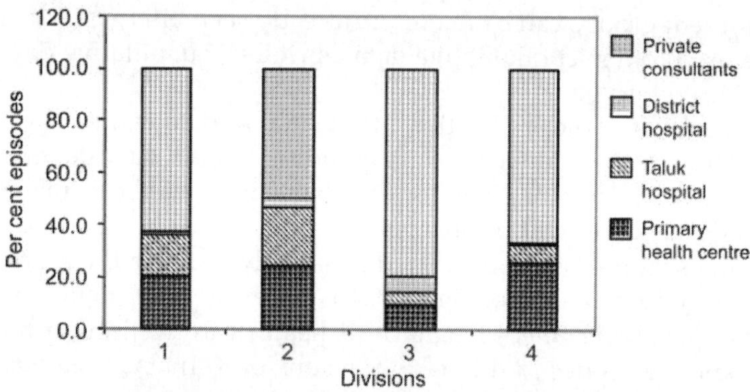

Fig. 6.5: Proportional bar diagram of place of OPD consultation for sickness in different divisions of Karnataka

v. Histogram

When quantitative data of continuous type is to be depicted in the form of a graph, histogram is useful. In drawing this graph, rectangles are erected as in the case of bar diagrams with its width equal to the class interval of the variable on the horizontal axis and the corresponding frequency on the vertical axis as its height. But unlike in bar diagrams, all the bars are drawn continuously, i.e. adjoining to each other.

The basic concept behind this graph is that the area under each rectangle, when taken as a proportion of the total area under all the rectangles, gives the probability of occurrence of the value of the variable, corresponding to the class interval covered under the base of that particular rectangle. If the total area is taken as one, then area under each rectangle represents the proportional probability for that class interval. This will be useful to compare the probability of occurrence of various values of the variable in the distribution.

Haemoglobin levels of students in a class are depicted as histogram in Figure 6.6.

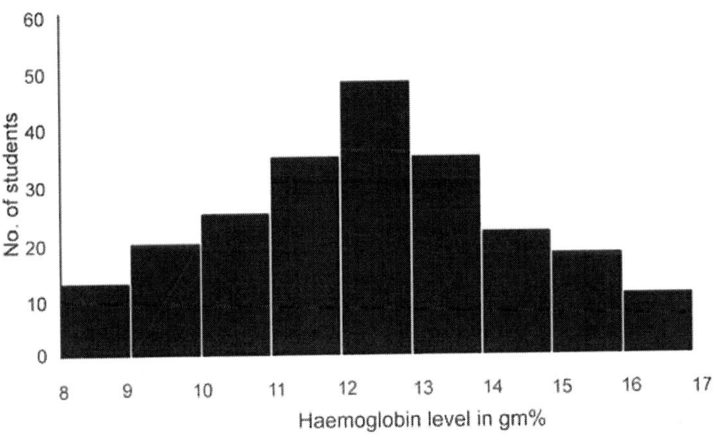

Fig. 6.6: Histogram showing the haemoglobin level of students in a class

vi. Frequency Polygon

This graph is useful to depict frequency distribution of quantitative data in the form of a curve. This is useful especially when it is necessary to compare two or more frequency distributions. The curves for different distributions are drawn with different shades of lines on the same graph paper for easy identification. Such comparisons will not be possible through histograms because the boundaries of the rectangle may overlap resulting in confusion.

While drawing these graphs, it is assumed that the frequencies corresponding to each class interval is equally distributed around the middle point of the class interval. As in the case of histograms, the values of the variables are marked on the horizontal axis and the frequencies on the vertical axis (Fig. 6.7). The frequency corresponding to each class interval is marked on the graph by a point corresponding to the location of middle point of class interval. Points corresponding to all the class intervals of the distribution are joined by a smooth line. The end points of the line are joined to the X-axis by joining the curve at the middle point of the previous class interval at the start and then at the end to the middle point of the next to the ultimate class interval of the distribution. This closing of the curve with the X-axis is done to make it a polygon and also to ensure that the total area under the curve is equal to the area of the corresponding histogram. In certain cases the line may have to be extended to the negative side which may be fallacious or in some other cases the values of the variable can never take the values beyond the range depicted in the table. Hence in such cases it is not advisable to join the curve to the base as described above, but is to be joined to the beginning class-interval and end point of the last class-interval.

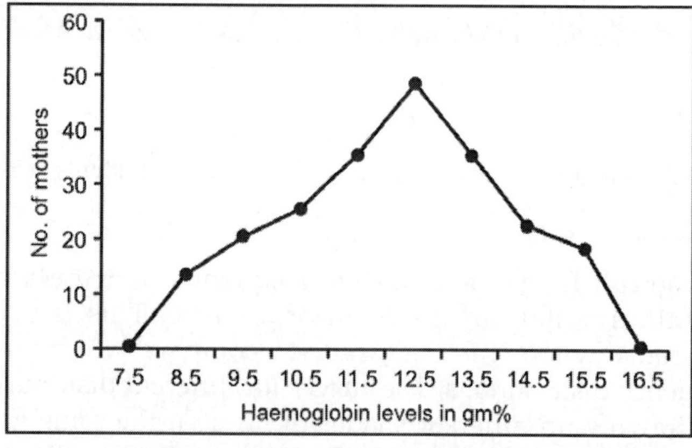

Fig. 6.7: Frequency polygon of haemoglobin levels of antenatal mothers in a community

When two or more distributions with marked difference in their frequencies are to be compared it will be more appropriate to plot the percentages rather than the actual frequencies.

vii. Pie Diagram

This graph is useful for depicting qualitative data. In this diagram a circle is divided into different sectors corresponding to the frequencies of the values of the variable. Each segment of the circle will be proportional to the frequency of the variable in the data. The segments correspond to the angle subtended by the segment at the centre of the circle.

Because the total angle at the centre of the circle is equal to 360° and since it represents the total frequency, the angle subtended at the centre for each segment for any value of the variable is given by the following formula :

Angle at the centre for any segment or group

$$= \frac{\text{Frequency in the specific group}}{\text{Total frequency in all the group}} \times 360°$$

After the calculation of the angle for each group, segments are marked off in the circle in succession corresponding to the angle at the centre for each segment. The segments are then shaded with distinctive shades or colours or numbered and a separate index is given for these shades or numbers.

In Figure 6.8, Pie diagram for place of treatment for OPD consultations in Karnataka State is depicted.

This graph is effective only when the number of groups are not many and the number of observations in each group can be added to get the total number of observations of all the values of the variables.

viii. Scatter Diagram or Correlation Chart

All the diagrams discussed in the previous paragraphs are useful only for frequency distribution with single variables. When two variables are observed on the same individual, sometimes it may become necessary to study the possible relationship between the two variables. In such cases scatter

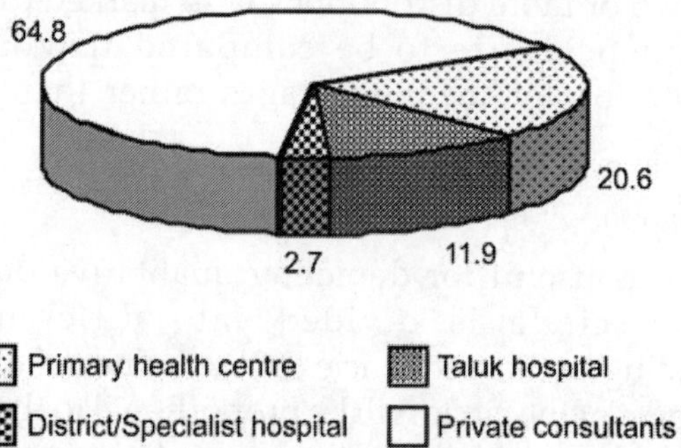

Fig. 6.8: Place of treatment for OPD consultations for sickness episodes in Karnataka state

diagram is used to interpret any relationship that may exist between the two variables (Fig. 6.9).

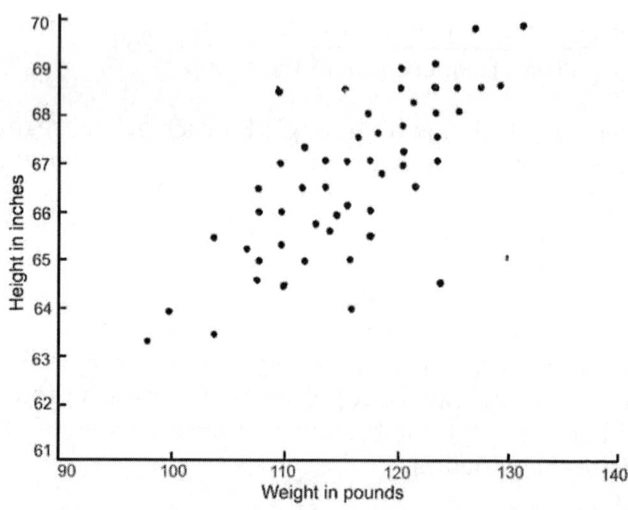

Fig. 6.9: Scatter diagram showing height and weight of male students in a class

In this graph the two variables are represented on the two axes of the graph paper. Then each point plotted on the graph will be corresponding to one set of observation of the two variables for each unit of observation. There will be as many points as there are pairs of observations. After plotting all the points, when they are viewed collectively the trend of the points will suggest any possible correlation that may exist between the two variables.

Further details of these graphs are given in chapter under Correlation and Regression.

ix. Age and Sex Pyramid

This graph is useful for depicting the age and sex pattern of a community (Fig. 6.10). In this graph two histograms are drawn on both sides of the vertical axis with their bases adjoining to each other with a common scale. One histogram corresponds to the age distribution of males and the other to that of the females.

Unlike in other histograms here the frequencies, i.e. the number of persons in any age group is taken on the horizontal axis and the variable, i.e. age groups, is taken on the vertical axis.

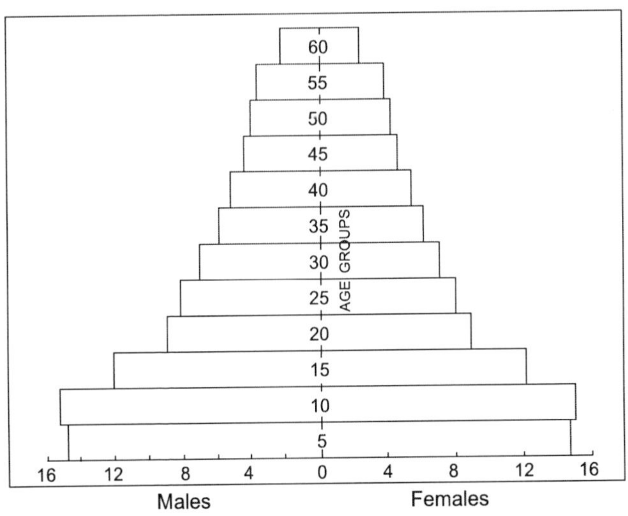

Fig. 6.10: Age and sex pyramid of a sample population in a survey

7 Chapter
Measures of Central Tendency

Need for Measures of Central Tendency

It was understood in the previous chapters that most of the observations in this universe are subject to variability and this is more predominant with biological observations. It is a known fact that the biological observations like those of weight, height, pulse beat per minute or blood counts of the groups with respect to persons with similar age, sex, health status, etc. differ from person to person. In order to make a sensible definition of the group or to identify the group with reference to the observations, it is required to express the observations in a precise manner. That is to say that the observations are to be expressed as a single estimates so that this estimate summarises the observations. This estimate is useful not only as a precise estimate of the series of data but also useful to compare two or more sets of data.

It was seen in Chapter 5, that a frequency distribution could be compared within itself in terms of the frequencies between various class intervals. Scope of comparing two or more distributions, in terms of different class intervals is very much limited. But when it is a question of overall comparison of the distributions, comparing them in terms of frequencies within class intervals is not advantageous and the only alternative way is to compare them in terms of a single estimate of the observations of the data.

Such estimates of the data of any distribution, which summarises the distribution, are known as the parameters of the distribution. These parameters define the distribution completely. One such parameter is the measure of Central Tendency.

As the name itself indicates it gives an estimate of the centre of the distribution.

The concept of centre may be different in different contexts. In one context it may be some mathematical estimate of the centre, while in the other, it may be the exact central observation in the order of magnitude or in another it may be the value of the observation with maximum frequencies. Based on these contexts three measures of central tendency have been defined.

These three measures of central tendency are : Mean, Median and Mode. Each of them has their application in different types of data and circumstances as discussed in subsequent paragraphs.

Definition and Calculation of Mean

Mean gives an estimate of the centre in terms of averages. The simplest average is the arithmetic average and in the common terminology, mean refers to this arithmetic average. Similarly there are other averages like geometric mean and harmonic mean. But mean, the arithmetic average has the highest utility in branch of statistics and so wherever the word mean occurs, unless specified otherwise, always refers to this arithmetic average.

Mean is calculated from the formula;

$$\text{Mean} = \frac{\text{Sum of all the observations of the data}}{\text{Number of observations in the data}}$$

Mean calculated for any sample is symbolically represented as

$\bar{x} = (\Sigma x_i) / n$

Where sigma, Σ, means the sum of,

$x_{i,}$ is the value of each observation in the data

n is the number of observations in the data

$\bar{x}$ is the symbol for mean.

Usually Σ_i is used to indicate the sum of all observations over the values of i. But for the sake of simplicity instead of Σ_i only Σ is used in the subsequent paragraphs and chapters.

Calculation of Mean for an Ungrouped Data

An ungrouped data has already been described as the data which is not classified into any table. In such a case the mean is calculated directly or through simplified method given below.

i. Direct Method

In this method the mean is calculated by first adding all the values of the observations and then dividing this sum by the number of observations.

Example 7.1. Systolic blood pressure in mmHg of ten students are as follows:

115, 117, 121, 120, 118, 122, 123, 116, 118, 120.

$$\text{Mean} = \frac{(115+117+121+120+118+122+123+116+118+120)}{10}$$

$$= (1190) / 10 = 119 \text{ mmHg}$$

ii. Alternative Method

If the values of the observations are large, in order to minimise the labour of additions, the size of the value of each observation can be reduced by subtracting a particular value of the observation. This value of the observation should be usually nearer to the actual mean and can be located by inspection of the observations. The value of the observation, which is subtracted from other values, is generally known as assumed mean.

After subtracting this assumed mean from other values, the observations are usually reduced to the form

.............-3, -2, -1, 0, 1, 2, 3..........,

Then the mean is calculated with new values as in the direct method. But the mean calculated thus has to be converted to the actual mean, which is obtained by the following formula.

Actual mean = Assumed Mean + (Sum of the new values/ No. of observations)

The term (Sum of the new values/No. of observations) can be called as the Correction Factor.

Example 7.2. For the data given in Example 7.1, by inspection, it may be assumed that the mean is around 120. Then 120 is subtracted from all the other values.

i.e. $115 - 120 = -5$
$117 - 120 = -3$
$121 - 120 = +1$
$120 - 120 = \ \ 0$
$118 - 120 = -2$
$122 - 120 = +2$
$123 - 120 = +3$
$116 - 120 = -4$
$118 - 120 = -2$
$120 - 120 = \ \ 0$

Now these new numbers are added and divided by 10 to get the correction factor.

$$\{(-5)+(-3)+1+0+(-2)+2+3+(-4)+(-2)+0\} / 10$$
$$= (-10) / 10 = (-1)$$

Actual mean = Assumed mean + Correction factor
= 120 + (–1) = 119 mmHg

It can be observed that the advantage of the above method lies in the simplification attained for the addition of big numbers.

Calculation of Mean for Grouped Data

When the number of observations are many, the above methods of calculation of mean will be laborious and hence the observations are to be grouped into frequency distribution table and the mean is to be calculated from this table. It can be recalled that in a frequency distribution table, the class intervals can be with either single value of the variable or with a group of values of the variable. Corresponding to these two methods of grouping, different ways of calculation of mean are available.

i. Grouped Data with Single Units for Class Intervals

a. Direct method

This method corresponds to the direct method of calculation of mean for ungrouped data.

In an ungrouped data, to get the sum of all the observations, each value of the observation is added once, but in a grouped data, the values are to be added as many times as the value occurs. In other words, each value of the variable is to be multiplied by its frequency of occurrence and all these products are then to be added to get the sum of all the observations. After getting the sum of observations in the above manner, it is divided by the number of observations to get the mean.

The formula for calculation of mean by this method is:

$\overline{x} = (\Sigma x_i f_i) / (\Sigma f_i)$

where x_i is the value of each grouped variable and f_i is the corresponding frequency and Σ refers to summation of values.

Example 7.3. For the distribution of number of illnesses of Table 5.1, the mean number of illness per individual in a year is obtained as follows.

No of illness x_i	No of individuals f_i	Product of (1) and (2) $x_i f_i$
0	24	0
1	76	76
2	114	228
3	115	345
4	86	344
5	51	255
6	26	156
7	18	126
Total	510	1530

$\Sigma x_i f_i = 1530$

$\Sigma f_i = 510$

Mean number of illness per individual in a year = $\overline{x}$

$= (1530 / 510) = 3.0$

b. Short-cut method or code method

Sometimes even though the variables measured may be tabulated in single units of class intervals, either the values of the variable may be large or the frequencies may be large. In such cases the product term will again be a huge number, which results in increased labour of addition besides the difficulty encountered in the multiplication of big numbers without a calculating machine. Hence in such a case the procedure is simplified by selecting an assumed mean of the values and calculating the mean as was done for ungrouped data.

This assumed mean of the value is subtracted from the values of the variable and thus their size is reduced. These new values are multiplied by the corresponding frequencies and their sum is divided by the number of observations. The actual mean is calculated as described in the case of ungrouped data by the following formula.

$$\bar{x} = x_c + [\{ \Sigma(x_i - x_c) f_i\} / (\Sigma f_i)]$$

where,

x_i is the tabulated value of the variable,

x_c is the assumed mean, which is subtracted from each of the above value of x_i,

f_i is the frequency corresponding to each x_i,

$(x_i - x_c)$ gives the new value obtained for each of the value of x_i after subtracting x_c.

Example 7.4. The following table gives the distribution of students according to their age. The mean age of the students is calculated as follows.

Age in years x_i	No. of students f_i	$(x_i - x_c)$	$(x_i - x_c) f_i$
(1)	(2)	(3)	(4)
16	72	–4	–288
17	155	–3	–465
18	302	–2	–604
19	496	–1	–496
20	546	0	0
21	660	+1	+660
22	455	+2	+910
23	332	+3	+996
24	191	+4	+764
25	109	+5	+545
Total	**3318**		**2022**

In the above example x_c is assumed as 20, and column (3) is obtained by subtracting 20 from each value of the age in column (1).

– 4 is obtained by subtracting 20 from 16,

– 3 is obtained by subtracting 20 from 17 and so on.

Column (4) is obtained by multiplying each of the values in column (3) by the frequencies by its side in column (2).

i.e., $-288 = -4 \times 72$

$-465 = -3 \times 155$

$-604 = -2 \times 302$ and so on

By adding all these products

$\Sigma (x_i - x_c) f_i = 2022$

Now, by substituting these values in the equation

$$\overline{x} = x_c + [\{\Sigma(x_i - x_c)f_i\} / (\Sigma f_i)]$$

Mean age of students = 20 + (2022 / 3318)

= 20 + 0.61

= 20.61 years

ii. Grouped Data with a Range for Class Intervals

a. Middle point method

When the range of the values of the variable is very wide, usually the values of the variable are grouped into appropriate class intervals and the corresponding frequencies are tabulated as a frequency distribution table.

In such cases, the mean is calculated from this frequency distribution table assuming that the frequencies in a class interval are uniformly distributed on both sides of the middle point of the class interval. By this assumption the calculation of the product of the frequency and variable is facilitated, because only the middle points of the class intervals will now be used instead of the class intervals themselves. Middle points are obtained as the average of upper limit and lower limit of the class interval.

With the middle points being considered the procedure for calculating the mean is similar to the direct method of grouped data with single units of class interval.

The mean is obtained from the formula.

$$\bar{x} = [(\Sigma x_i f_i) / (\Sigma f_i)]$$

Where x_i is the middle point of the class interval and f_i is the frequency in the class interval and Σ refers to summation of values.

Example 7.5. For the data of Hb% levels of a sample of individuals, the mean Hb% level is calculated as follows.

Hb. in gm%	Middle point of class interval x_i	Frequency f_i	$x_i f_i$
(1)	(2)	(3)	(4)
9.1-10.0	9.55	10	95.50
10.1-11.0	10.55	21	221.55
11.1-12.0	11.55	67	773.85
12.1-13.0	12.55	170	2133.50
13.1-14.0	13.55	84	1138.20
14.1-15.0	14.55	29	421.95
15.1-16.0	15.55	4	62.20
Total		**385**	**4846.75**

The procedure for the calculation of mean of the above data is as follows:

Middle points in column 2 are obtained as

$(9.1 + 10.0) / 2 = 9.55$

$(10.1+11.0) / 2 = 10.55$ and so on,

column (4) gives the product of the middle points in column (2) and the corresponding frequencies in column (3).

Thus the sum of the products in column (4) will be

$$(\Sigma x_i f_i) = 4846.75$$

and the sum of the frequencies in column (3) is $(\Sigma f_i) = 385$

Mean $= \bar{x} = [(\Sigma x_i f_i) / (\Sigma f_i)] = (4846.75 / 385) = 12.59$ gms %.

b. Alternative method

It may be observed from the previous example, that it will be difficult, without using a calculator, to multiply the middle point and the frequency when either or both of them are big numbers or when the middle points are in decimals.

To facilitate multiplication, the alternative method given in the case of grouped data with single units can be applied, when all the class intervals are of the same size.

Firstly, the assumed mean value in terms of the middle points is located. Then this value is subtracted from each of the middle point of the class interval and then these new values are divided by their common factor, i.e. the size of the class interval. In other words, the procedure is that the new value will be zero for the middle point corresponding to the assumed mean and all the middle points higher than the assumed mean will have numbers +1, +2, +3,........ and lower ones will be –1, –2, –3 and so on.

These new values are multiplied by the corresponding frequencies and then the sum of these products is obtained.

This sum is divided by the number of observations to get the mean according to these new values. Actual mean is obtained by multiplying this value by the length of the class interval.

Actual mean is obtained by the formula,

$$\overline{x} = x_{do} + [(\sum f_i d_i \times l) / (\sum f_i)]$$

where x_{do} = middle point corresponding to the zero of the new value

d_i = new values of the middle points

f_i = frequencies corresponding to each middle point

l = length of the class interval.

It is to be noted that this method is useful only when all the class intervals are of the same size.

Example 7.6 The calculation of the mean Hb% level for the data given in the Example 7.5 by this method is as follows.

Hb. level in gm%	Middle points of class interval	Frequency	New values for middle points	
	x_i	f_i	d_i	f_id_i
(1)	(2)	(3)	(4)	(5)
9.1-10.0	9.55	10	–3	–30
10.1-11.0	10.55	21	–2	–42
11.1-12.0	11.55	67	–1	–67
12.1-13.0	12.55	170	0	0
13.1-14.0	13.55	84	+1	+84
14.1-15.0	14.55	29	+2	+58
15.1-16.0	15.55	4	+3	+12
Total		**385**		**15**

In column (4) it may be seen that the new value corresponding to the middle point 12.55 is substituted as zero. This is done so because maximum number of frequencies are there in this class interval and as such the mean may be somewhere near this middle point. The other middle points higher than this have been given the values 1, 2, 3, while the lower ones are replaced by –1, –2, –3, since the length of the class interval is unity.

Thus the calculated values are:

$$\Sigma f_i d_i = (154 - 139) = 15$$

$$\Sigma f_i = 385$$

$$l = \text{length of the class interval} = 1.0$$

$$x_{do} = 12.55$$

By substituting these values in the formula we get

$$\begin{aligned}\bar{x} &= (12.55) + (15/385) \times 1.0 \\ &= (12.55) + (0.04 \times 1.0) \\ &= 12.59 \text{ gm\%}\end{aligned}$$

Meaning and Interpretation of Median

It was seen that the mean is the arithmetic average of the observations. It is needless to say that average depends upon the size of the individual observations from which they are calculated. If there are a few observations which are quite extreme in their magnitude and which are quite away from most of the observations the value of the mean is either inflated or deflated according to the deviations of the extreme observations.

As an example, if the period of stay of patients in a ward of hospital is considered, majority of the patients might have stayed in the ward for treatment from 1 to 15 days but in a few cases it may happen that they have stayed for one or two months. If the mean is calculated taking all these periods into consideration the value of the mean will be very high which may be far from the central value of observation.

Hence the mean as a measure of central tendency, in this type of observations, is fallacious. In such cases the best estimate of the centre would be to locate the magnitude of the exact central observation.

This estimate of the centre is known as Median. In other words the median is that value of the variable or observation which divides the series of observations into two equal halves according to the magnitude of the variable.

The application of median in the field of medicine can be illustrated by another example. In measuring the dose response in pharmacology in order to know the effect of several doses of a drug, it is customary to calculate the median lethal dose or median response dose. This measurement gives that particular concentration or the dose of a drug, which kills exactly 50% of the animals or is toxic to 50% of the animals respectively.

However, when the frequency distributions are symmetrical, and when there are not many observations deviating from the central value on either side, the median value will not differ much from the mean.

Calculation of the Median

i. Ungrouped Data

For a data, which is not grouped, the median is calculated by arranging all the observations in the order of their magnitude and then selecting the value of the middle observation. When the number of observations are odd it is easy to select the middle observation but when the number of observations are even, the average of the values of the middle two observations will be the median.

Example 7.7. In a hospital ward the following are the number of days of stay of patients.

13, 42, 8, 9, 7, 3, 6, 52, 8, 2, 11, 11, 10, 9.

For the calculation of the median all the numbers are first arranged in the order of their magnitude.

2, 3, 6, 7, 8, 8, 9, 9, 10, 11, 11, 13, 42, 52.

As there are 14 patients, the average of the period of stay corresponding to the 7th and 8th patients is calculated as the median.

i.e. Median = (9+9) / 2 = 9

ii. Grouped Data

When the data consists of many observations, it is laborious to arrange all of them in ascending or descending order and then to locate the middle observation. In such cases it will be easier to arrange the data into a frequency distribution table and to calculate the median from this table.

As already understood, in a frequency distribution table the values of the variable are already in an ascending order, either as a single unit or as a class interval with the corresponding frequencies. Hence it may be taken that the values are all arranged in the order of their magnitude.

If an additional column giving the total frequencies upto each of the class interval is included in the table, which can be obtained by adding all the frequencies up to and above that particular class interval, it will be easy to locate class interval in which middle observation is contained. The total of the frequencies up to a class interval calculated in the above manner is known as the *Cumulative frequency* and the distribution of such frequencies for the different class intervals is known as the *Cumulative frequency distribution.*

The class interval in which the middle observation is contained is located by inspection of these cumulative frequencies.

After locating this class interval, the median value is calculated by the formula,

Median = L_i + [{ (N/2 - f′) (i) / (f_{med})}]

N is replaced by (N+1) if number of observations is even.

Where L_i, is the end value of the class interval previous to the median class interval.

f_{med} is the frequency in the class interval in which the median is located which is known as median class interval.

f′ is the cumulative frequency of the class interval previous to the median class interval.

N is the total number of frequencies.

i is the length of the median class interval.

When N, the total number of frequencies is sufficiently large it will not be wrong to take the value of N/2nd observation as the frequency corresponding to the median value, whether the number of observations is even or odd.

Example 7.8. Going back to the example of Hb% levels of previous examples, the median for the data can be calculated as follows.

Hb level in gm%	Frequency	Cumulative frequency
(1)	(2)	(3)
9.1 - 10.0	10	10
10.1 - 11.0	21	31
11.1 - 12.0	67	98
12.1 - 13.0	170	268
13.1 - 14.0	84	352
14.1 - 15.0	29	381
15.1 - 16.0	4	385
Total	**385**	

Total number of observations = 385

Observation corresponding the middle

or median value = 385/2 = 192.5

It can be seen from column (3) of cumulative frequencies 192.5th observation is located in the class interval 12.1 to 13.0 as 98 observations are up to Hb% level 12 gm% and 268 frequencies are up to 13 gm%.

Thus, $f_{med} = 170$

$L_i = 12.0$

$f' = 98$

$N = 385$

$i = 1$ gm%

$$\text{Median} = 12.0 + \{(192.5 - 98) / 170\} \times 1$$

$$= 12.0 + (94.5 / 170) = 12.0 + 0.56 = 12.56 \text{ gm\%}$$

iii. Graphical Method for Locating the Median

The median can also be located from the curve obtained by plotting the cumulative frequencies against the end points of the corresponding class intervals as shown in Figure 7.1, which is the data corresponding to frequency distribution of haemoglobin level of 385 individuals of above example. This curve is known as *Ogive*. The curve is plotted by taking the variable on the X-axis and the cumulative frequency on the Y-axis.

To locate the median from the curve the following procedure is adopted.

On the Y-axis the point corresponding to the N/2nd frequency is located and from this point, a line parallel to X-axis is drawn to meet the curve. At the point of this intersection, a line parallel to Y-axis is drawn to meet the X-axis. The value corresponding to the point of intersection of this line on the X-axis is the median value of the observations.

As is seen from Figure 7.1, the total frequency is 385, and the N/2th frequency is 192.5.

Corresponding to this point 192.5 on the Y-axis, a line parallel to X-axis is drawn to meet the curve. From this point again a line parallel to Y-axis is drawn to meet the X-axis. The value corresponding to this point is 12.56, which is the median value of the series of observations.

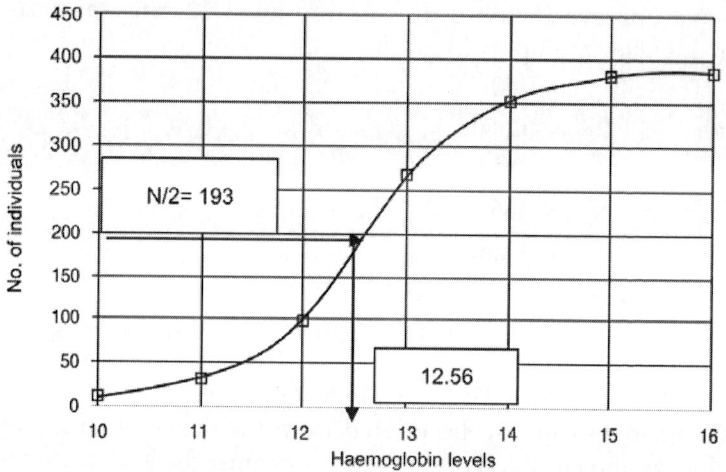

Fig. 7.1: Curve obtained by plotting the cumulative frequencies against the end points of the corresponding class intervals (Ogive).

Meaning and Calculation of Mode

Another measure of central tendency, which is less influenced by the value of the individual observation, is the mode. This corresponds to that value of the observation, which has highest frequency. In other words mode can be defined as the most common value of the observation.

The mode is more useful in certain type of observations where it is required to know the value of the observation, which has high influence in the series.

As an example, when studying the age of onset of a disease it is desirable to know the age at which the maximum number of persons are affected rather than the mean age of onset or median age of onset.

The mode is located from the frequency distribution table, taking the value of the variable with maximum frequency.

In the Example 7.4, the mode for the data on the age of students, is 21 years as there are maximum number of students with that value of the variable.

It is also to be noted that in a frequency polygon, the mode can be located from the point where the curve takes a turn from increase to the decrease. There can be more than one mode for a series of data.

Mode can also be calculated from the relationship:

Mode = Mean – 3 (Mean – Median).

8 Chapter

Measures of Dispersion and Skewness

Need for Measures of Dispersion

In the previous chapter, it was understood that one of the parameters useful for defining a distribution in a concise manner is the measure of central tendency. But by knowing only the mean, median or mode it is not possible to fix the distribution completely. For example, if there are two groups of families, one with their family sizes as 2, 2, 3, 5, 5, 5, 7, 8, 8, and the other with 3, 3, 3, 3, 5, 5, 6, 7, 10, it can be seen that both the groups of families have their mean and median size as 5. But at the same time it can also be seen that most of the family sizes of the two groups are different. Hence two sets of data with a common mean or median need not be same with regard to the various individual values of the observations.

Hence it is essential to know how far these observations are scattered from each other or from the mean. Measures of these scatter or variation are known as *Measures of dispersion or variation*. By knowing these measures of dispersion along with the measures of central tendency, most of the biological distributions can be completely defined and thereby they can be easily compared with each other.

Like different measures of central tendency, there are different measures of variation. But each of them have their merits and demerits and are used in different circumstances.

The most common measures of dispersion are:

(i) Range
(ii) Mean deviation
(iii) Standard deviation
(iv) Coefficient of variation.

Range

In the example given in Table 7.1, in addition to the mean or median or modal values, sometimes it is interesting to know as to what is the minimum and the maximum systolic blood pressure. It can be seen from the data that the systolic blood pressure ranges between 115 to 123. In other words the minimum and maximum values of the variable are noted for these cases. This measure of the scatter of the values of the variable is known as the Range. The range thus gives the values of the two extreme observations of the variable, however, range does not provide any information about the other values in the series of data.

This method is simple to comprehend as well as to calculate but is useful only on certain occasions. Range is misleading when the extreme values are of unusual occurrence.

Some times instead of knowing the range between all the observations, we may be interested to know the range within which a certain percentage of observations lies. Such a range is called as *Percentile range*. Suppose, if we note down the value of the variable covering up to the first 25 per cent of the observations, it is called as 25th percentile (Q_1). Similarly the value of the variable covering upto the first 75 per cent of observations is called as 75th percentile (Q_3). Incidentally it may be noted that median is the 50th percentile value of the variable. These three values of the variables are also known as *Quartiles* as they divide the distribution into quarters.

Another measure of dispersion based on the values of quartiles is the quartile deviation or the semi interquartile deviation, Q.

It is calculated as $Q = (Q_3 - Q_1) / 2$

Mean Deviation

It is always better to find the deviation of the individual observations with reference to a certain value in the series of observations and then to take an average of these deviations. This deviation is usually measured from mean or median but mean is more commonly used for this measurement. The index of variation is known as the Mean Deviation or Average Deviation.

Thus the mean deviation about the mean can be defined as the average of the absolute value of the deviations between the mean and each of the values of observation in the series and is calculated by the following procedure.

First the mean of the observation is calculated. Then the mean is subtracted from each of the observations. The mean of these deviations is then calculated by averaging all these deviations without considering the sign of the deviation, which gives mean deviation.

Mathematically it is written as,

$$MD = (\Sigma | (x_i - \bar{x}) |) / n$$

where MD refers to mean deviation:

x_i refer to individual values of the observations

$\bar{x}$ is the mean

n is the number of observations

and | | refers to the absolute value and termed as modulus

Example 8.1. The mean deviation of the data of systolic blood pressure given in Example 7.1 is calculated as follows:

x_i	$(x_i - \bar{x})$
115	115 – 119 = – 4
117	117 – 119 = – 2
121	121 – 119 = + 2
120	120 – 119 = + 1
118	118 – 119 = – 1
122	122 – 119 = + 3
123	123 – 119 = + 4
116	116 – 119 = – 3
118	118 – 119 = – 1
120	120 – 119 = + 1

$(\Sigma (| x_i - \bar{x} |) = 22$

$MD = (\Sigma | (x_i - \bar{x}) |) / n = 22 / 10 = 2.2$

Incidentally, it may be noted that $\Sigma (x_i - \bar{x})$, i.e. the sum of deviations taking signs into consideration is zero and hence the absolute values of these differences are taken.

In a grouped data mean deviation is calculated using the formula:

$$MD = [\Sigma (\mid (x_i - \bar{x}) \; f_i \mid] / n$$

Where x_i refers to the middle point of the class interval and f_i is the frequency in the class interval. The other symbols are having the usual meaning.

Standard Deviation

In the calculation of mean deviation, the signs of the deviation of the observation from the mean were not taken into consideration. In order to avoid this discrepancy, instead of the actual values of the deviations, if the squares of the deviations are considered for calculation, a quantity known as *Variance* can be calculated by averaging the squares of the above deviations. Square root of the variance is considered as a measure of variation of the observations, the square root of variance is known as *Standard Deviation.*

In other words, Standard deviation is the square root of the mean of the squared deviations of the individual observations from the mean. It is also called as *Root Mean Square Deviation.*

Of all the different measures of dispersion, standard deviation is the most important one and it is mostly used in various statistical methodologies described later. It is one of the important parameters of the standard distributions like normal and some of the skewed distributions, which will be discussed in Chapter 9.

Further, standard deviation is useful in tests of significance or in measurement of correlation between two sets of data and various other statistical analysis.

It is conventional to represent the standard deviation of a sample by, s, and that of a population by σ and it is expressed in the same unit as that of original observations.

Calculation of Standard Deviation

The Standard Deviation (SD) of any data is calculated from the basic formula:

$$\sigma = \sqrt{[\{(\Sigma (x_i - \bar{x})^2\} / n]}$$

Where x_i is the value of each observation,
$\bar{x}$ is the mean value and
n is the number of observations.
Σ refers to summation

For the calculation of the estimate of the standard deviation of the original population from which the sample has come out, the standard deviation is calculated from the following formula:

$$s = \sqrt{[\{(\Sigma (x_i - \bar{x})^2\} / (n - 1)]}$$

As we usually require the estimate of the standard deviation of the original population, s, is taken as the best estimate of σ and hence it is customary to calculate the standard deviation from the above formula.

i. Calculation of Standard Deviation for an Ungrouped Data

a. Direct method

The steps involved in the calculations are as follows:

The mean $\bar{x}$ of the observations is calculated,

The deviation of each of the observation in the sample from the mean i.e. $(x_i - \bar{x})$ is computed.

Squares of these deviations are tabulated,

Sum of these squares i.e. $\Sigma (x_i - \bar{x})^2$ is obtained,

This sum $\Sigma (x_i - \bar{x})^2$ is divided by (n -1), where n is the number of observations to get the variance.

The square root of variance is worked out to get the standard deviation.

Example 8.2. The pulse rates per minute of 10 students in a class are as follows:

80, 90, 96, 80, 94, 72, 84, 92, 82, 90.

The standard deviation of the pulse rate for the group is calculated as below:

	x_i	$(x_i - \bar{x})$	$(x_i - \bar{x})^2$
	80	80 – 86 = –6	36
	90	90 – 86 = +4	16
	96	96 – 86 = +10	100
	80	80 – 86 = –6	36
	94	94 – 86 = +8	64
	72	72 – 86 = –14	196
	84	84 – 86 = –2	4
	92	92 – 86 = +6	36
	82	82 – 86 = –4	16
	90	90 – 86 = +4	16
Total	**860**		**520**

$$\text{Mean} = \bar{x} = (\Sigma x_i) / n = 860 / 10 = 86$$

$$\Sigma (x_i - \bar{x})^2 = 520, \qquad n = 10$$

$$s = \sqrt{[\{(\Sigma (x_i - \bar{x})^2\}/(n-1)]}$$

$$s = \sqrt{(520/9)}$$

$$= \sqrt{(57.78)} = 7.60 \text{ per min.}$$

b. Alternative method

Sometimes it may be difficult and laborious to take the difference in each case and to take the square of these deviations. As a simplification it may be easier to take the squares of the individual observations themselves. In such cases standard deviation can be calculated from the formula:

$$s = \sqrt{[\{\Sigma x_i^2 - (\Sigma x_i)^2 / n\} / (n-1)]}$$

The steps involved in this method are:

Sum of all the observations is obtained and this sum is squared to get $(\Sigma x_i)^2$.

This $(\Sigma x_i)^2$ is divided by n, the number of observation to get $(\Sigma x_i)^2 / n$

Each observation is squared and the sum of these squares is obtained to get Σx_i^2

These quantities are substituted in the given formula and standard deviation is obtained.

Example 8.3. The size of a group of 10 families are 3, 3, 4, 7, 8, 12, 6, 5, 4, 4 and the standard deviation is calculated by the above method as follows.

x_i = 3, 3, 4, 7, 8, 12, 6, 5, 4, 4

Σx_i = 56

x_i^2 = 9, 9, 16, 49, 64, 144, 36, 25, 16, 16

Σx_i^2 = 384

$(\Sigma x_i)^2 = (56)^2 = 3136$

$(\Sigma x_i)^2/n = 3136/10 = 313.6$

$[\Sigma x_i^2 - (\Sigma x_i)^2 / n] = (384.0 - 313.6) = 70.4$

$$s = \sqrt{[\{\Sigma x_i^2 - (\Sigma x_i)^2/n\} / (n - 1)]}$$

$$= \sqrt{(70.4 / 9)} = \sqrt{(7.82)} = 2.8$$

ii. Calculation of Standard Deviation for Grouped Data

As seen already, when the number of observations is large, usually, the data will be grouped into a frequency distribution table either with single units or a group of units for class interval. In such cases the standard deviation is calculated by the following method.

a. Method for class interval with single units

In this case the Standard deviation is calculated from the formula;

$$s = \sqrt{[\{\Sigma (x_i - \bar{x})^2 f_i\} / (n - 1)]}$$

Where, x_i is the value of individual observation.

f_i is the frequency corresponding to each x_i,

$\bar{x}$ is the mean and

n is the number of observations.

Example 8.4. For the data of number of illnesses per individual of Example 7.3, Standard deviation is calculated as follows:

No. of illness x_i	No. of individuals f_i	$x_i f_i$	$(x_i - \bar{x})$	$(x_i - \bar{x})^2$	$(x_i - \bar{x})^2 f_i$
0	24	0	–3	9	216
1	76	76	–2	4	304
2	114	228	–1	1	114
3	115	345	0	0	0
4	86	344	+1	1	86
5	51	255	+2	4	204
6	26	156	+3	9	234
7	18	126	+4	16	288
Total	**510**	**1530**			**1446**

$$\bar{x} = (\Sigma x_i f_i) / n = (1530) / 510 = 3.0$$

$$\{\Sigma (x_i - \bar{x})^2 f_i\} = 1446$$

$$s = \sqrt{[\{\Sigma (x_i - \bar{x})^2 f_i\} / (n - 1)]}$$

$$= \sqrt{(1446 / 509)} = \sqrt{2.84} = 1.69$$

b. Alternative method

As seen in the alternative method for calculation for ungrouped data, standard deviation can be calculated by taking the squares of the observations directly instead of taking the squares of the differences of the value of the observation and the mean.

$$SD = \sqrt{[\{ (\Sigma x_i^2 f_i) - (\Sigma x_i f_i)^2 / n)\} / (n - 1)]}$$

Where, x_i, f_i and n have their usual meaning.

Example 8.5. For the data of the previous example, the standard deviation is calculated by the above method as follows.

No. of illness per individual x_i	No. of individuals f_i	$x_i f_i$	x_i^2	$x_i^2 f_i$
0	24	0	0	0
1	76	76	1	76
2	114	228	4	456
3	115	345	9	1035
4	86	344	16	1376
5	51	255	25	1275
6	26	156	36	936
7	18	126	49	882
Total	**510**	**1530**		**6036**

$\Sigma x_i f_i = 1530$

$\Sigma x_i^2 f_i = 6036$

$n = \Sigma f_i = 510$

$(\Sigma x_i f_i)^2 = (1530)^2 = 2340900$

$(\Sigma x_i f_i)^2 / n = 2340900 / 510$

$= 4590$

By substituting the above values in the formula

$$s = \sqrt{[\{(\Sigma x_i^2 f_i) - (\Sigma x_i f_i)^2 / n)\} / (n - 1)]}$$

$$s = \sqrt{\{(6036 - 4590) / 509\}}$$

$$= \sqrt{\{1446 / 509\}}$$

$$= \sqrt{\{2.84\}} = 1.69$$

c. Calculation for grouped data with a range for class intervals

When the class intervals are in terms of a range, then as in the case of the mean, it is assumed that the frequencies are all centred a round the middle points of the class intervals. These middle points are substituted for the values of the variable x_i for each range of class interval and the standard deviation is calculated by any of the above two methods.

Example 8.6. The following data gives the number of eosinophil per 100 WBC counts in a unit volume of blood as detected during the health examination of students.

The calculation of standard deviation is illustrated below.

No. of eosinophil per 100 WBC count	Middle points of class intervals x_i	No.of students f_i	$x_i f_i$	x_i^2	$x_i^2 f_i$
0-4	2	409	818	4	1636
5-9	7	101	707	49	4949
10-14	12	21	252	144	3024
15-19	17	9	153	289	2601
20-24	22	3	66	484	1452
25-29	27	2	54	729	1458
30-34	32	2	64	1024	2048
45-49	47	2	94	2209	4418
Total		**549**	**2208**		**21586**

Where, n = 549

$\Sigma x_i f_i = 2208$

$(\Sigma x_i f_i)^2 = 4875264$

$(\Sigma x_i f_i)^2 / n = 4875264 / 549$

$= 8880.2$

$\Sigma x_i^2 f_i = 21586$

By substituting the above values in the formula

$$s = \sqrt{\{(21586.0 - 8880.2)/548)\}}$$

$$= \sqrt{(12705.8/548)}$$

$$= \sqrt{(23.186)} = 4.82$$

d. Short-cut method or code method

As in the case of calculation of mean, in order to simplify the calculations, the code method can be used when the length of all the class intervals are same. Procedure for substituting of codes in place of middle points is same as described for the calculation of the mean. The standard deviation is then calculated with the codes in place of the middle points.

In order to get the actual standard deviation, the standard deviation obtained with codes is to be multiplied by the length of class interval.

Mathematically it can be written as:

$$s = \sqrt{[\{\Sigma (d_i^2 \times f_i) - (\Sigma d_i f_i)^2 / n\} / (n - 1)]} \times (1)$$

Where d_i is the code for each class interval

f_i is the frequency in each class interval

n is the number of observations

1 is the length of the class interval

It may be noted here that the standard deviation does not depend upon the origin of the calculation.

Example 8.7. The standard deviation of the haemoglobin level of students in a class is calculated as follows.

Hb in gm%	Mid point of class interval	Frequency f_i	Codes for mid points d_i	$d_i f_i$	d_i^2	$d_i^2 f_i$
9.1-10.0	9.55	10	–3	–30	9	90
10.1-11.0	10.55	21	–2	–42	4	84
11.1-12.0	11.55	67	–1	–67	1	67
12.1-13.0	12.55	170	0	0	0	0
13.1-14.0	13.55	84	+1	84	1	84
14.1-15.0	14.55	29	+2	58	4	116
15.1-16.0	15.55	4	+3	12	9	36
Total		**385**		**15**		**477**

$$\Sigma d_i^2 f_i = 477$$

$$\Sigma d_i f_i = 15$$

$$(\Sigma d_i f_i)^2 = (15)^2 = 225$$

$$(\Sigma d_i f_i)^2 / n = 225/385 = 0.58$$

$$n = 385 \text{ or } (n-1) = 384$$

SD according to code

$$s = \sqrt{[(477 - 0.58) / 384]}$$

$$= \sqrt{[(476.42) / 384]}$$

$$= \sqrt{(1.2407)} = 1.11$$

Actual SD = (SD according to code) × (length of the class interval)

$$= 1.11 \times 1.0$$

$$= 1.11$$

Measures of Relative Deviation

When the deviation of observations within a series is to be measured, the standard deviation is the best measure. But the size of the standard deviation depends upon the size of the mean as well as the unit of measurement of observation. Hence to compare the variations of two or more variables which are in different units as well as with marked difference in the size of the means, comparison with standard deviation is not suitable.

As an example, the variation of the haemoglobin level of a group of students and variation of their body weights will have different means and they are measured in different units. Haemoglobin level is expressed as gm % while the body weight will be in kilograms, further the size of the mean haemoglobin level will be smaller while the mean body weight will be a big number and the size of the standard deviations will also be different.

In order to compare the deviations of such variables of data, the standard deviation is expressed as a percentage to the mean value and this quantity is known as *Coefficient of Variation*. This has no unit but it is expressed as a percentage.

Mathematically,
Coefficient of Variation = (Standard Deviation x 100) / Mean

Calculation of the coefficient of variation is illustrated in the following example.

Example 8.8. The mean and standard deviation of the haemoglobin level of a group is 12.6 gm% and 1.5 gm% respectively while the mean and standard deviation of the body weight of the same group is 50 kg and 2.2 kg respectively.

To compare the deviations of these two sets of observations coefficient of variation is calculated for each of the data.

Coefficient of variation of Hb level = (1.5 / 12.6) x 100
= 11.9%

Coefficient of variation of body weight = (2.2 / 50) x 100
= 4.4%

From these values it can be seen that the variation is greater for haemoglobin level than for body weight of the group although the absolute value of standard deviation was higher for body weight.

Skewness

When a frequency distribution or a frequency curve is not symmetrical about the peak, it is said to be skewed. In other words one tail of the curve will be longer than the other in a skewed curve. This skewness can be either to the right or left of the peak.

A relative measure of skewness given by Karl Pearson is :

Skewness $= 3(\bar{x} - \text{Median}) / s$

Where, $\bar{x}$ is the mean, and s is the standard deviation of the distribution.

When this calculated quantity is positive it indicates that the skewness is to the right and when it is negative it indicates skewness to the left, when it is zero, there is no skewness.

Chapter 9 Probability and Standard Distributions

Meaning of Probability

Probability is a common word used in day to day life meaning some chance factor for the occurrence of any specified event, such as the chances of a person winning a lottery or chances of a particular operation being successful and so on. Thus the probability is a certain mathematical quantity which depends upon the quantum of occurrence of either favourable or unfavourable cases affecting the occurrence of an event. This quantity is in fact a ratio of two numbers, i.e. the quantity obtained by dividing one number by another number.

The probability of an event can be defined as the ratio of the number of favourable cases for the particular event to the total number of cases both favourable and unfavourable to this event. As an example consider the event of enumerating the persons who had an attack of a disease in a community. The probability of coming across a person with the history of an attack of the disease is the ratio of the number of persons with the history of attack of the disease to the total number of persons in the community.

As another example, if the probability of a patient leaving the hospital against medical advice during a year's time is to be computed, then this will be the ratio of the number of patients who have left the hospital against medical advice during a year's time to the total number of patients admitted to the hospital during that year.

If the total admission to the hospital during a year is say 'N' and out of whom 'n' number of patients left the hospital against medical advice then the probability of any patient leaving the hospital against medical advice, denoted P (A) is equal to (n/N).

Thus probability of an event

$$= \frac{\text{No. of favourable cases for the event}}{\text{Total number of cases both favourable as well as unfavourable to the event}}$$

Example 9.1 Suppose in a class there are 100 students out of whom 90 are boys and 10 are girls. Then the probability of a student chosen at random out of the students in the class to be a girl is

$$= \frac{\text{No. of girls in the class}}{\text{Total no. of both boys and girls in the class}}$$

$$= \frac{10}{100} = 0.1$$

Probability can have a lowest value of *zero* and a highest value of *one* according to the number of favourable cases for the event. In other words, according to the value of the numerator, when the numerator is zero, i.e. none of the cases are favourable for an event out of the total cases, then the probability of the event will be zero. When all the cases are favourable for the event, both the numerator and the denominator will be equal and hence the probability of that event will be one.

In the above example, if there are no girls in the class and all the students are boys then the probability of a student chosen at random to be a girl is zero and the probability of a student chosen at random to be a boy is one.

When there are only two complimentary events of occurrence then the probability of a particular event will be equal to (1- probability of the other event).

As can be seen from example 9.1, the probability of selecting a boy at random

= 90/100 = 0.9

= (1 – Probability of selecting a girl)

For most of the variables, the probability of occurrence of a particular event attains more and more consistency when the variable is enumerated in large numbers. For example, the probability of a new born being a boy will be almost equal to 0.5 when a large number of births are enumerated. This type of consistent probability for any event is a common feature of many of the biological variables.

From the theory of probability, models for the distribution of biological data have been formulated and this is the basis of all statistical hypotheses. These distributions are described in further paragraphs.

Standard Distributions

Most of the variables when classified into a frequency distribution follow a certain fixed pattern. This pattern becomes more and more consistent with the increase in the number of observations. That is to say, that when a biological variable is measured or enumerated on sufficiently large number of observations and the frequency distribution of these measurements are plotted, the curve tends to take a particular shape. This shape will be similar for a particular variable if repeated observations are made in large numbers. The shape of the curve may be different for different variables. The shape of these curves are governed by certain mathematical laws based on the probability of occurrence of different values of the variable. The probability of occurrence of different values of observations can be depicted in terms of these mathematical laws. These laws are known as *probability distribution laws* of the variable. From these distributions the number or the percentage of observations lying at a particular value of observation or up to or beyond a value can be estimated. In any frequency distribution, if the frequencies are plotted against the values of the variable, the area under the curve up to any value of the variable is a function of the cumulative probability of occurrence of that particular value of the variable. So when the exact probability distribution law of any variable is known, the shape of the curve, the probability of occurrence of various values of observations, etc. can be determined, as discussed in subsequent paragraphs.

The three fundamental standard probability distributions of importance in the statistical theory are discussed in the following paragraphs in the order of their importance.

Normal Distribution

This distribution is the most important one in biological observations and is common to many of the biological variables, when observed in large numbers.

Suppose if the values of haemoglobin levels of a large number of individuals are enumerated and plotted on a graph paper in the form of a histogram or a frequency polygon, it can be observed from the graph, that there would be maximum number of observations corresponding to the centre of the curve, the number of observations gradually decrease on both sides of this point with very few observations at the tail ends and further the curve would be symmetrical. This type of distribution is known as *Normal distribution* (Fig. 9.1).

The mathematical equation of this distribution is

$$y = \{1/ \sigma \sqrt{(2 \pi)}\}\ e^{-\frac{1}{2}\{(x_i - \mu)/\sigma\}^2}$$

where, y is the frequency corresponding to the variable value of x_i

μ is the mean value of the variable in the population

σ is the standard deviation of the variable in the population

π is the mathematical constant with value 3.4159.......

e is the mathematical constant, 2.71828...., the base of natural logarithms.

Usually μ and σ are estimated from the samples and these estimates are represented as $\bar{x}$ and s respectively.

The following are the important characteristics of Normal Distribution.

i. The shape of the distribution resembles a bell.

ii. The curve is symmetrical about the middle point.

iii. At the centre of the distribution which is peaked, all the three measures of central tendency namely the mean, median and mode coincide.

iv. Maximum number of observations are at the value of the variable corresponding to the mean and the number of observations on both sides of this value gradually decrease and there are only a few observations at the extreme points.

v. The area under the curve between any two points which corresponds to the number of observations between any two values of the variable can be calculated in terms of a relationship between the mean and the standard deviation.

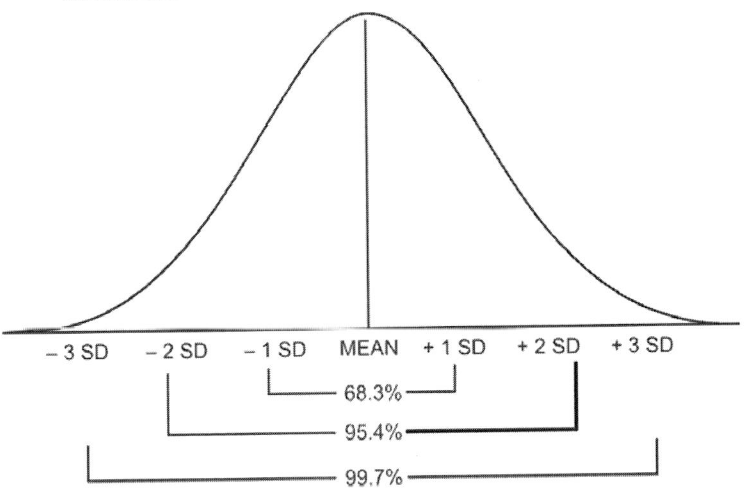

Fig. 9.1: Normal distribution curve

The three simple relationships are :

a. (Mean ± 1 SD) covers 68.3% of the observations.
b. (Mean ± 2 SD) covers 95.4% of the observations.
c. (Mean ± 3 SD) covers 99.7% of the observations.

Thus from the above relationship it can be seen that almost all the values of the observations lie within the range of (Mean ± 3 SD) and most of the values of the observations are within the range of (Mean ± 2 SD). This relationship is useful for fixing the confidence intervals of the statistical parameters.

vi. Normal distribution law is the basic assumption for various tests of significance.

Standard Normal Variate

When a variable x follows a normal distribution with mean $\overline{x}$ and standard deviation s, then the quantity,

$$Z = \{(x - \overline{x}) / s\}$$

is known as the *Standard Normal Variate* (SNV). The values of Z for several values of x follows a normal distribution with a mean value equal to *zero* and a standard deviation *one*.

All variables following a normal distribution pattern with any mean and standard deviation can be transformed to a Standardised Normal Variate using the above formula. This quantity facilitates the calculation of proportion of the frequency of observations between any two values of the variable or up to or beyond a value of the variable, with the help of Normal probability integral table (Appendix Table 1), irrespective of the values of mean and standard deviation of the original observations.

Similarly when the mean and standard deviation of a variable following a Normal distribution is known, the probability of occurrence of any of the variable can be calculated from the above table. In this Normal probability integral table, the area of the Normal curve up to a particular value of SNV from + ∞ or - ∞ is tabulated. As the curve is symmetrical the values are tabulated for only one half of the curve.

The practical applications of above procedures are illustrated in the following examples.

Example 9.2. If the body temperature of healthy persons in a community is distributed normally with a mean 37° C, and standard deviation 0.3° C, then the proportion of persons with a body temperature 37.5° C or above is calculated as follows.

First the SNV is calculated for the given value of the variable from the formula. From Appendix table 1, the probability level corresponding to this calculated value is noted. This tabulated value gives the probability for the variable having a value from maximum of $+\infty$ up to the given value of the variable. This probability when multiplied by 100 gives the percentage population beyond the value of the variable.

Here $x = 37.5°$ C, $\bar{x} = 37.0°$ C, $s = 0.3°$ C

$$(x - \bar{x}) = (37.5 - 37.0) = 0.5$$

$$Z = \{((x - \bar{x}) / s\} = (0.5 / 0.3) = 1.67$$

The area of the curve beyond this point as seen from the Appendix table 1 is 0.04746. This corresponds to the probability that the variable takes a value 37.5° C or above.

In other words (0.04746 x 100) or 4.75% of the healthy population have their body temperature of 37.5° C or above.

Example 9.3. In the above example, if the problem is to find the proportion of persons in the population within a range of body temperature 36.5° C to 37.5° C, the procedure is as follows:

In this case the two SNVs corresponding to the above values of the variables are calculated and the proportion of areas of the curve for the values of the variable below the lower value and above the higher value are calculated from the Appendix Table 1. By adding these two proportions, the total proportion of the area of the curve below and above two desired values of the variable is obtained which when multiplied by 100 gives the percentage of persons in the population with the body temperature beyond 36.5° C and 37.5° C. By subtracting this proportion from 100, we can obtain the proportion of persons with body temperature in the range 36.5° C to 37.5° C.

It is worked out as follows.

$x_1 = 36.5°$ C, $\bar{x} = 37.0°$ C, $s = 0.3°$ C

$$(x_1 - \bar{x}) = (36.5 - 37.0) = -0.5$$

$$Z_1 = (-0.5 / 0.3) = -1.67$$

$x_2 = 37.5°$ C, $\bar{x} = 37.0°$ C, $s = 0.3°$ C

$$(x_2 - \bar{x}) = (37.5 - 37.0) = +0.5$$

$$Z_2 = (+0.5 / 0.3) = +1.67$$

The proportion of the area under the curve from $-\infty$ upto $-1.67 = 0.04746$.

Here the negative sign indicates the left-hand side of the curve.

The proportion of the area under the curve from $+\infty$ upto $+1.67 = 0.04746$.

The proportion of the area under the curve beyond these two points = $(Z_1 + Z_2)$.

= (0.04746 + 0.04746) = 0.09492 or 0.095 or 9.5 percent

Therefore the percentage of persons between the two values of the body temperatures.

= (100 – 9.5) = 90.5%

In other words, in the population there would be 90.5% of persons with body temperature between 36.5° C to 37.5° C.

Binomial Distribution

When the population under observation can be divided into two distinct groups, one with a certain characteristic and the rest without this characteristic, the distribution of the occurrence of the characteristic in the population is defined by the Binomial Distribution.

As an example, in a given population, if it is required to define the distribution of prevalence of a certain disease, then the entire population can be divided into two groups, one with the disease and the other without the disease. If the probability of a person having the disease is p and not having the disease is q, i.e., (1–p), then the distribution of various probabilities, i.e. the probability of finding none, one, two, three, four,.... persons with the disease in a group of n persons is given by the successive terms of the binomial distribution $(q+p)^n$

The expansion of $(q+p)^n$ is given by the formula,

$$(q+p)^n = q^n + {}^nC_1\, q^{n-1} p + {}^nC_2\, q^{n-2} p^2 + {}^nC_3\, q^{n-3} p^3 + \ldots\ldots + {}^nC_r\, q^{n-r} p^r + \ldots\ldots + {}^nC_{n-1}\, q\, p^{n-1} + p^n$$

$$= \sum_{r=0}^{n} {}^{n}C_{r} q^{n-r} p^{r}$$

Where ${}^{n}C_{r}$ = n! / (r! (n–r)!)

n! means, factorial n = n(n–1)(n–2) .... 2 × 1

and r! = r(r–1)(r–2) .... 2 × 1

${}^{n}C_{r}$ denotes the number of combinations of *r* things taken at a time out of *n* things.

In the above expansion, the first term q^n gives the probability that none of the persons in the group of n persons is suffering from the disease while the second, third .... rth .... (n+1)th term gives the probability that one, two, three ....(r-1)...n persons are suffering from the disease respectively. Hence the probability that at most 1, 2, ... r .... n persons are suffering from the disease is given by the sum of the successive 1st, 2nd, 3rd, .. (n+1)th terms of the above expansion respectively.

Actual frequencies are obtained by multiplying these probabilities by the number of groups observed.

Example 9.4. In a community if the probability of a person with any disease on any day is 0.1, then the corresponding probability that a person is not suffering from the disease is 0.9.

Then in a house of six members the probability that none, one, two, three, four, five and all six persons are having the disease on any day is given by the successive terms of the expansion.

$(0.9+0.1)^6 = (0.9)^6 + {}^{6}C_{1}\,(0.9)^5\,(0.1)^1 + {}^{6}C_{2}\,(0.9)^4\,(0.1)^2 + {}^{6}C_{3}(0.9)^3(0.1)^3 + {}^{6}C_{4}(0.9)^2(0.1)^4 + {}^{6}C_{5}(0.9)(0.1)^5 + (0.1)^6$.

The probability that in the family of 6 persons, no person is sick on any day

$= (0.9)^6 = 0.531441.$

The probability that in the family of 6 persons, 1 person is sick on any day.

$$= {}^6C_1\ (0.9)^5\ (0.1) = \frac{(6!)}{(1!)\ (5!)}\quad \{(0.9)^5\ (0.1)^1\}$$

$$= \frac{(6 \times 5 \times 4 \times 3 \times 2 \times 1)\ \{(0.9)^5\ (0.1)^1\}}{(1) \times (5\times4\times3\times2\times1)}$$

$$= 6\ (0.9)^5\ (0.1)^1$$

$$= 6\ (0.59049)\ (0.1)$$

$$= 6\ (0.059049)$$

$$= 0.354294 \text{ or } 0.35$$

Similarly the probability that in the family of 6 persons, 2 persons are sick on any day

$$= {}^6C_2\ \ (0.9)^4\ (0.1)^2$$

$$= \frac{(6!)}{(2!)\ (4!)}\quad \{(0.9)^4\ (0.1)^2\}$$

$$= \frac{(6\times5\times4\times3\times2\times1)\ \{(0.9)^4\ (0.1)^2\}}{(2\times1)\ (4\times3\times2\times1)}$$

$$= 15\ (0.6561)\ (0.01)$$

$$= 15\ (0.006561)$$

$$= 0.098415$$

If we observe 100 such households then the number of households with none, one, two persons suffering from the disease is the number obtained by multiplying each of the above terms by 100, i.e., 53, 35 and 10.

Thus the number of households with a maximum of two persons sick on any day is given by the sum of above products of the first three terms as illustrated below.

No. of households out of 100 houses with a size of 6 persons

with none sick at any time = $(0.531441 \times 100) = 53$
with one person sick at any time = $(0.354294 \times 100) = 35$
with two persons sick at any time = $(0.098415 \times 100) = 10$

Hence No. of houses with a maximum of two persons sick = (53+35+10) = 98

Main Characteristics of the Distribution

In a binomial distribution,

i. Mean number of events with the characteristic is given by (np) where n is the number of observations and p is the probability of occurrence of the characteristic.
ii. Variance of the number of events is (npq) where q = (1–p).
iii. If p and q are equal, i.e. each equal to 0.5, the curve will be symmetrical.
iv. If p and q are not equal then the curve will be skewed.
v. For any fixed value of p and q, if n, i.e. the number of observations is increased to a sufficiently large size, binomial distribution becomes more and more symmetrical and tends to be a normal distribution.

Poisson Distribution

If in a binomial distribution, the value of p or q becomes infinitely small and n, the number of observations becomes very large so that the product (np), the mean number of events is always finite, then the binomial distribution tends to be a Poisson distribution. Here the occurrence of an event at any point of time is independent of previous event.

In this distribution the probabilities of the event occurring 0, 1, 2, 3 ... r times is given by the successive terms of the exponential series

$$e^{-m}\left(1+m+\frac{m^2}{(2!)}+\frac{m^3}{(3!)}+\ldots\ldots\ldots\ldots\right)$$

where e refers to the base of natural logarithms,
m mean number of events
! is factorial as described earlier.

Suppose in a surgical ward the post-operative management is quite efficient, then the number of deaths due to post-operative management will be quite small and as such the probability of deaths due to post-operative complications on any day will be quite low. To estimate the probability of the number of days with no death, one death or two deaths and so on, in a year's time, due to post-operative management, Poisson distribution can be utilised.

First the mean number of deaths per day is calculated out of the data for a certain period and this mean (m) is substituted in the above formula to estimate the various terms in the series.

The probability of (r) number of deaths on a day is given by the (r+1)th term of the above series. The number of days with r number of deaths in a year is obtained by multiplying this probability by 365.

If it is required to estimate the number of days with at most r deaths, then the estimated days up to 0, 1, 2, ... r deaths are to be added or the total probability of up to r deaths is to be multiplied by 365.

The following example will illustrate an application of Poisson distribution in the health care management.

Example 9.5. In a big hospital, it was observed from previous records, that the number of post-operative deaths in year's period was 60. Number of days with no post-operative death, or the number of days in a year with one or two post-operative deaths can be calculated as follows, using Poisson distribution.

m = Mean number of post-operative deaths per day in a year's period

$$= \frac{\text{Number of post-operative deaths in a year}}{\text{No. of days in the year}}$$

$$= 60/365 = 0.16438$$

Using this Mean the probability of none, one or two deaths on any day can be calculated through successive terms of the Poisson distribution

$$e^{-m}\left(1 + m + \frac{m^2}{(2!)} + \frac{m^3}{(3!)} + \ldots\ldots\ldots\right)$$

Probability of number of deaths per day can be calculated as follows.

No death $= e^{-m}\ (1) = e^{-0.16438} = 0.84842$

One death= $(e^{-m})\ m = (e^{-0.16438}) \times (0.16438)$

$= (0.84842) \times (0.16438)$

$= 0.1395$

Two deaths $= \dfrac{m^2 (e^{-m})}{(2!)} = \dfrac{(0.16438)^2 (0.84842)}{2 \times 1}$

$= 0.01146$

The number of days in a year with none, one, two deaths can be calculated by multiplying these probabilities by 365, i.e. No. of days in a year with *no deaths*=(0.84842 × 365)
= 310 days

One death = (0.1395 × 365) = 50 days
Two deaths = (0.01146 × 365) = 4 days

Thus there will be almost negligible number of days with three or more deaths.

Main Characteristic of the Distribution

In a Poisson distribution

i) Mcan = m
ii) Variance = mean
iii) The distribution can be defined in terms of the mean only.

10 Chapter
Sampling Techniques

Necessity and Meaning of Sample

The object of all investigations is to secure some information and also to make comparisons with similar available data. It was learnt in the previous chapters that from a mass of data one can make comparisons using the parameters like mean, standard deviation, etc. calculated for the data. On the one hand, such data is collected by experimentation in clinical medicine while on the other, some of the health data is obtained through permanent health agencies set up for the purpose like the data on births, certain diseases suffered by the community, etc. But such data collected are neither complete nor will mean anything unless they are viewed in the background of various other factors like sociological, biological, economical, administrative and several other factors. In other words they are to be analysed in the light of epidemiological and etiological factors concerned with the causation of the phenomenon. To obtain such information it will not be practicable to carry on the investigation with each and every person in the community. Usually they are obtained from a smaller group of the community, selected to represent the entire population depending upon the available resources, precision and nature of the data required. Even in clinical experimentation the investigations are carried out on a smaller group of patients or animals to get the knowledge on the entire group. The method of selecting such smaller groups and other aspects of sampling are discussed in the subsequent paragraphs.

Before proceeding further, firstly the meaning of some words like *population* or *universe* and *sample*, which we often come across, are to be understood.

The word population or universe means an aggregate of units of observation either animate or inanimate about which certain information is required. Thus, when recording the pulse rate of boys in a college, all boys in the college constitute the population or universe. When studying the houses in a town according to the incidence of a certain disease, all the houses in the town constitute the population. When experiments are conducted on human beings or animals, such human beings or animals constitute the population.

The word sample means a portion or a part of the above population selected in some manner. Thus a sample for the first population mentioned above is a specified number of boys out of all the boys in the college while a sample for the second population means a specified number of houses out of all the houses in the town.

When the investigation is carried out for the entire population it is called as the census enumeration and when it is carried out for the sample it is called a sample enumeration.

Criteria for a Good Sample

A sample can be selected broadly in two ways. One method is by selecting only those units of the population so that it suits a specific purpose as per the desire of the investigator and a sample selected by this method is known as a *Purposive sample*. This method of selection serves a very limited purpose. The other method is by selecting the units of the sample in such a manner that the characteristics of the population is represented in the sample. This is possible by selecting the units of the sample at random. A sample so selected is called as *Random sample or Probability sample*. In this method of sampling each unit included in the sample will have a certain pre-assigned probability of inclusion in the sample.

Reliable and accurate generalisations about the population are possible only through random samples and not through purposive samples. All statistical techniques can be applied only to random samples. Another advantage of the random sample is that it takes care of all biases, which may or may not occur during investigations.

Some Applications of Sampling in Community Health

Sampling is very useful in all the investigations on community health as complete enumeration of the community may not be always possible. A few of the common applications are mentioned below.

i) *Evaluation of Health Status of a Population*

As already indicated, the health status of a community is expressed in terms of several health indicators. The data for such indicators will be obtained through random sample surveys of the community, by collecting the general information regarding the disease prevalent in a community and their associated epidemiological factors. Surveys can also be for special sicknesses such as tuberculosis, trachoma, filariasis or nutritional deficiencies or any other health factor. These surveys will help in assessing the incidence or prevalence rates and other epidemiological aspects of the diseases.

Sample surveys are also conducted to know the demographic data of the community such as age and sex structure, sex ratio and other sociological data.

For knowing the incidence rates of the disease and some other follow up particulars, longitudinal sample surveys are conducted.

ii) *Investigations of Factors Influencing Health*

For effective control of any disease mere prevalence or incidence data will not be useful unless they are viewed in the light of other factors responsible for the causation of the disease such as environment, nutrition, genetic background and such other factors. Such etiological information are obtained through sample surveys. Surveys on knowledge, attitude and practices (KAP) regarding health are also examples of some of the investigative surveys which are carried out on random samples.

iii) *Studies on Environmental Hygiene*

Sample surveys are useful in certain environmental studies such as estimation of extent of contamination of water, estimation of degree of adulteration of food, etc. Such surveys are similar to quality control in industries.

In surveys of this type, usually a standard for contamination will be fixed and samples are examined to find out whether the contamination is above or below the fixed standard. The population from which the samples have come out will be judged as contaminated or not, depending upon the results obtained from the sample.

Such conclusions are very useful in judging the quality of food consumed by the community as it will not be possible to examine each and every individual's consumption in a community.

iv) *Studies on the Evaluation of Health Measures*

Sample surveys are useful to estimate the effect of health measures such as control of tuberculosis or malaria or effectiveness of health education programmes, etc.

v) *Studies on the Administrative Aspects of Health Services*

Several health data relating to health facilities for planning and extension of health programmes in the community are collected through sample surveys. Information such as availability and extent of usage of medical facilities can be obtained by sample surveys from door to door survey or sample analysis of hospital and dispensary records.

vi) *Advance Data from Surveys*

To get advance information from survey data or to check the accuracy of the data collected, sample surveys are useful. Random subsamples of the entire sample can be used for such purposes.

Census Enumeration Versus Sampling Enumeration

Census enumeration	Sampling enumeration
1. All units are covered and information will be available for each unit of the universe.	Only specified units are covered and information will be available for only those units which are in the sample.
2. Useful when detailed information is required for each unit of the population.	Useful when overall information about the population is required.
3. Cost of organisation and enumeration will be more.	Cost of organisation and enumeration will be less as the sample will not be as large as the population.
4. Greater attention cannot be paid for each unit because of the vastness of the population.	Greater attention can be paid to each unit in the sample and only a few specially trained people are required for the collection of information due to the relative smallness of the sample.
5. Will be difficult to achieve completeness and accuracy.	Completeness and accuracy can be achieved by more persistent efforts.
6. Requires more personnel and time both for collection and analysis.	Requires less personnel and time for collection and analysis.

Method of Selecting a Random Sample

Usually random samples are selected using *Random Number Tables*. Specimen of these tables are given in Appendix Table 2. The procedure for selecting a random sample is as follows.

First the unit of selection is decided. The unit may be a village, a household or an individual in a community or in a drug trial, the animals or patients to be included for the study, etc. Then all these units are arranged in some suitable order either in the alphabetical order of names or chronological order and so on and numbered serially. This is known as the *sampling frame*. The number of units to be included in the sample is fixed on the basis of the factors discussed in the subsequent paragraphs. Then the serial number of the units to be included in the sample are obtained as detailed below.

A random number table is chosen and within it a row and a column is selected at random. At the point of intersection of the selected row and column, as many columns are clubbed together as there are number of digits in the total population size. That is to say that if there are up to 99 units in the population two columns are clubbed together, if there are up to 999 units in the population, three columns are clubbed together. Then after such clubbing, the numbers in the list starting from this point are read downwards and all numbers less than or equal to the total number of units in the population are noted down. When the last row of these columns is reached then a corresponding number of columns next to them is taken and the procedure is repeated. All the duplicate numbers are deleted and the selection is continued till the desired size of the sample is obtained. The selected numbers correspond to the serial numbers in the list of the population and these units constitute the sample.

Example 10.1. To select a random sample of 25 students from a class of 75 students.

i. In this case the unit of selection is a student. Hence all the 75 students in the class are arranged in some order say alphabetical order of their names and they are numbered from 1 to 75.

ii. From Appendix Table 2, it is seen that there are 50 columns of single digit numbers in each table. Out of these a row and a column are selected at random. Say the 8th row and the 6th column are selected. The number corresponding to the intersection of this row and column is 6.

iii. The total population size is 75 and hence two adjacent columns are to be clubbed together, i.e. column 6 and 7 are clubbed together and is read as two digit numbers.

Now the number at this point of starting corresponds to 61.

iv. Starting from this number 61, the other numbers are read downwards and all numbers less than or equal to 75 are noted down.

v. When the last row of these columns 6 and 7 is reached the numbers from the top of the columns 8 and 9 are read down-wards as above and the procedure is repeated till 25 unduplicated numbers are obtained.

The numbers so read are

61, 62, 02, 31, 51, 11, 56, 64, 21, 01, 16, 39, 06, 38, 26, 34, 08, 65, 22, 52, 07, 29, 30, 14, 18

vi. The students corresponding to the above serial numbers constitute the sample. It is advisable to carry on the investigations in the same order of the numbers selected to ensure randomness even if the investigation is stopped before completing all the selected units.

Sampling Designs

Several sampling designs are available depending upon the type and nature of the population as well as the objectives of the investigation. A few of the important designs are given below:

i. *Simple Random Sampling*

In this method of sampling, a sample of say 'n' units out of 'N' units in the population is selected so that all the units in the population have an equal chance or probability of being included in the sample. As already described, the sampling units may be human beings, animals or any other objects depending upon the investigation. This method of sampling can be applied when the parameter to be estimated is homogeneously distributed in the population and sampling frame for the universe is available.

For the purpose of selection, all the 'N' units in the population are arranged in some unbiased order and are serially numbered. Then a sample of 'n' numbers is selected out of these 'N' numbers at random as described in the previous paragraphs.

As an example, to select a simple random sample of 25 students from a class of 75 students, the following procedure is adopted.

All the roll number of the 75 students are considered as the sampling frame. Then 25 unduplicated numbers less than or equal to 75 are selected at random as detailed earlier and the roll number of the students specified forms a simple random sample.

ii. *Stratified Random Sampling*

In this method of sampling the entire population is divided into certain subgroups depending upon the characteristics to be studied and random samples are drawn independently from each of the subgroups. These subgroups are known as 'strata'.

This type of sampling is used when the population is heterogeneous with regard to the characteristics under study. That is to say, when the characteristic which is to be estimated from the sample is different with different subgroups of the population and these subgroups are not equally constituted in the population, then this type of sampling is designed to reduce the variance of the estimated value of the characteristics. In such types of population, homogenous subgroups are formed out of the population and samples are drawn from each of the subgroups separately. As an example, if it is known that the prevalence of a certain disease is different in different age groups then to estimate the prevalence rate of the disease from the sample, the survey is carried out taking stratified random sample from each of the age groups of the population, as the number of people in each age group is not equal in the population.

By this type of stratified sampling procedure, the precision of estimate of the characteristics under study is increased, and also due representation of the population is maintained. Advantage of this type of sampling is that the estimates of the characteristics under study can be made for each strata separately.

iii. *Systematic Random Sampling*

In this method of sampling the first unit of the sample is selected at random and the subsequent units are selected in a systematic way as the name itself indicates. If there are 'N' units in the population and 'n' units are to be selected for the sample, then 'N' is divided by 'n' and if 'q' is the quotient and 'r' is the reminder obtained after this division, then one number less than or equal to the reminder i.e. *'r'* is selected at random. This will be the first unit in the sample. The other units are obtained by the addition of this quotient 'q' to the previously selected number in a sequential manner. This 'q' is known as the *sampling interval.* If the reminder is *zero,* then one random number is selected out of the quotient itself and the procedure is repeated as described above.

The above procedure is followed when the total size of the population is known and the other particulars of the units are not known. This type of sampling can also be adopted in cases of selecting samples out of patients attending a clinic or dispensary and when the sampling frame cannot be prepared in advance. As a simple illustration, this sampling is similar to that of selecting every alternate patient or to select every fourth or fifth patient who attends the clinic, after selecting the first patient at random. In this case nothing will be known about the selected patients in advance.

As another example of a field study, suppose if there are 210 villages in a Community development block and if it is desired to select 40 villages out of them, then 210 is divided by 40 and the quotient and the remainder will be 5 and 10 respectively. Then a random number will be selected out of 10, say 6 and this will be the first number to be included in the sample. Then 5 is added to this and so 11 will be the second number. Again 5 is added to this, so 16 will be the third number and so on.

Hence the serial numbers of the villages selected will be 6, 11, 16, 21, 26, 31 and so on up to 40 numbers.

This sample procedure is not valid if there is any periodicity of occurrence of particular event in the population, which may effect the result of the study.

iv. *Multistage Sampling*

In this type of sampling, sampling units are selected at various stages. As an illustration, if the prevalence of a disease is to be estimated in an area, first a sample of villages may be selected at random in the first stage, and out of these selected villages a random sample of houses can be selected in the second stage and out of these sampled houses a random sample of individuals may be selected in the third stage. The sampling designs may be either same or different at each stage.

The principle advantage of this type of sampling is that it permits the available resources to be concentrated on a limited number of units of the frame, which results in a lower cost per unit of the inquiry. Further this type of sampling design will reduce the cost of preparing a complete sampling frame, since detailed sampling frame has to be made only for the final stage.

Some of the disadvantages of this method of sampling are that the sampling error is usually increased as the variability between the ultimate sampling units will be lesser within the same section of the frame as compared to between the sections. Further due to the fact that the sampling units will usually be of unequal size at various stages with respect to the number included in the ultimate sampling units, estimation procedures involve providing proper weights to the size of universe at different stages.

Size of the Sample

An usual question, which is to be answered, while conducting an investigation will be about the size of the sample or in other words the number of units to be included in the sample. Bigger the sample better will be the precision of the estimates. But due weight is to be given for the time, cost as well as practicability of investigating a big sample. Hence always an optimum size of the sample, keeping in view of the above factors, is to be considered.

The estimation of sample size involves the following factors:

i) An approximate idea of the estimate of the characteristic under observation, as well as the variability of this characteristic from unit to unit in the population is required. This information can be usually obtained either from previous investigations or from a pilot investigation before the investigation is started. When we are interested in assessing the cure rate of a drug, it can be seen that if the cure rate is high then the effect of the drug can be measured from a small sample while if the cure rate is low then a bigger sample is required. This is reverse with the quantum of variability of the cure rate from unit to unit.

ii. An initial knowledge of the accuracy of the estimate of the characteristic desired from the investigation is also essential to estimate the sample size. This means that one should decide in advance as to what should be the maximum permissible error that can be allowed in the estimates to be obtained from the sample. If this error can be large then a small sample can serve the purpose. If this error has to be a small quantity, then bigger samples are to be selected for the investigation. This precision depends upon the purpose of the investigation as well as the decision that follows from the results.

iii. The probability level within which the desired precision of estimates is to be maintained is also a criterion for fixing the sample size. It can be easily perceived that higher this probability bigger should be the sample size.

iv. The availability of the experimental material, resources and other practical considerations also determine the size of the sample. Depending on these factors the criteria mentioned under (ii) and (iii) are to be suitably moderated and sample sizes are to be fixed.

From the above considerations it will be clear that the sample size is to be determined as an absolute number and not as a fraction of the population size. A sample of size 100 from a population of 10,000 (i.e. 1%) will provide almost the same information about the characteristic under study as a sample of the same size, i.e. 100 will provide from the same population of 1000 (i.e. 10%). The estimates of the mean or the variability required for the estimation of an adequate sample size are to be obtained from previous investigations. In the absence of such information, a preliminary inquiry has to be conducted to obtain such information.

In some situations like field surveys involving many variables greater accuracy may be required for estimates of some of the variables than those of certain others. In such cases one has to go in for multiphase surveys wherein a smaller sample would suffice for those information requiring lesser accuracy and bigger samples for those requiring greater accuracy.

In a stratified random sampling design the allocation of total sample size to different strata is carried out either in proportion to different strata size or in proportion to variability within each strata or by optimisation of variability within each strata and cost of enumeration in the respective strata.

Calculation of Sample Size for Field Surveys

a. When it is a field survey to estimate the prevalence rate of a disease the sample size is calculated by the formula.

$$n = (4pq/L^2)$$

Where n is the required sample size, p is the approximate prevalence rate of the disease for which the survey is being conducted. The knowledge of this is to be obtained from previous surveys or from a pilot survey and $q = (1 - p)$

L is the permissible error in the estimate of p.

The above formula has been worked out for a probability level of $P = 0.05$. That is to say that the prevalence rate p, estimated from the above sample size will have an error of L and is true in 95 out of 100 samples. However, the estimated sample size is to be appropriately increased taking into account of the design effect.

Example 10.2 In a community survey to estimate the prevalence rate of malnutrition amongst children, if it is assumed that the prevalence rate is about 40% then the sample size required to estimate the real prevalence rate of malnutrition amongst children with 5% error in estimated prevalence rate and with a probability of 0.05 not exceeding this error limit is calculated as follows:

$$
\begin{aligned}
p &= 40\% \\
q &= (100\text{-}40\ ) = 60\% \\
L &= 5\% \text{ of } 40\% = 2\% \\
n &= (4 \times 40 \times 60) / (2^2) \\
&= (4 \times 40 \times 60) / 4 \\
&= 2400
\end{aligned}
$$

2,400 children are to be examined to estimate the malnutrition amongst children with 5% error.

If we increase the error percentage to 10% depending upon our resources then,

$$
\begin{aligned}
L &= 10\% \text{ of } 40\% = 4 \\
n &= (4 \times 40 \times 60) / 16 \\
&= 600
\end{aligned}
$$

Only 600 children are to be examined to estimate the malnutrition amongst children with an error of 10%.

a) When conducting investigations to obtain information on quantitative data, the sample size is calculated by the formula.

$$n = (t_\alpha^{\,2} \times s^2) / e^2$$

where n is the desired sample size

s is the standard deviation of observations

e is the permissible error in the estimation of mean difference

t_α is the value of 't' statistic at α level from 't' tables.

Example 10.3 In a community survey to estimate the haemoglobin level of antenatal mothers, if it is assumed from pilot studies, that the mean Hb % level is about 12 gm % with a standard deviation of 1.5 gm % then the sample size required to estimate the Hb. Level with a permissible error of 0.5 gm% is obtained as follows:

$$s = 1.5 \text{ gm}$$
$$e = 0.5 \text{ gm}$$

t_α can be taken as 2, as it is conventional to use 5% level of significance.

$$n = \{2^2 \times (1.5)^2\}/(0.5^2)$$
$$= (4 \times 2.25)/(0.25)$$
$$= 36 \text{ antenatal mothers}$$

Errors in Sampling

Errors that can come up in a sampling investigation are of two kinds. They are sampling errors and non-sampling errors.

Sampling errors are due to faulty sampling design or small size of the sample. These errors can be reduced and estimated through sampling techniques.

The non-sampling errors are as follows:

i. *Coverage Errors*

These errors crop up when all the units in the sample are not covered due to non-response or non co-operation.

ii. *Observational Errors*

These errors are due to interviewer's bias or due to imperfect experimental techniques or an interaction of the above factors.

iii. *Processing Errors*

These are due to theoretical errors in statistical analysis or clerical errors or computational errors.

Above non-sampling errors can be reduced by intensive effort to get complete coverage of the units in the sample. Even after this if some units are not covered, either a sub sample of the non-respondents can be covered and the results of this sub sample may be applied to the non-response group as a whole or a substitution of similar individuals can be made in place of the non-response group. Interviewers bias or experimental errors can be reduced by setting up standards of interview of experimental techniques and by intensive training of the workers. Processing errors can be controlled by administrative control.

11

Chapter

Design of Clinical Trials

Meaning of Clinical Trials

The main aim of a clinical trial is to make comparisons between one type of treatment with another. The parameters of these comparisons may be just in terms of certain physiological or biochemical estimates or may be in terms of number cured under different treatment groups. Such comparisons need some careful thinking as well as scientific preplanning. A lot of variability exists within or between biological observations and this is even more predominant amongst clinical data. The effect of treatment for various diseases is not the same. As such the *Controlled clinical trials* play an important role in clinical experimentation.

The term controlled trail means conducting experiments on groups, which are formed in such a way that the different experimental groups are identical in all relevant aspects, except for the treatments they receive, to facilitate comparisons in a scientific way. Out of these groups all the groups may receive different treatments which are to be compared between themselves or one group may receive only a placebo while the remaining groups receive different treatments and the effect of the various treatments are compared against the effect of placebo.

The ultimate aim of all such controlled trials is to ensure enhanced preciseness in results and to get maximum information out of the experiments in most convincing manner. The planning aspect of controlled trials is to form such identical groups and to allot various treatments to these groups in an unbiased manner.

Principles to be adopted in Clinical Trials

Of the three basic principle of controlled clinical trials, the first one is the *Principle of Randomisation* meaning that the treatments are allocated to different units randomly, which provides better estimate of experimental error and takes care of extraneous variability. Randomisation ensures certain probability of allocation of treatments to different experimental units, which enables for the application of different statistical methodologies for inferring from the data. The second is the *Principle of Replication* which means that Experiments should be repeated with more than one group or treatment is applied on many units or subgroups instead of one, which increases the precision of the study. The third is the *Principle of local control,* which means that the total experimental group is divided into different homogeneous groups or blocks and the treatments are randomly assigned to these parts. This principle enables elimination of variability due to extraneous factors.

Types of Controls

There are various types of controls and their merits and demerits are detailed below:

a. Retrospective Control

In this method of comparison, a group of patients treated for a particular disease with a new drug by the experimenter are compared with the results of a group of patients of the same disease treated with any other drug in the past by the same or some other worker. No doubt this method of comparison reduces the labour of treating a group again with the drug already established for its efficacy but has its own discrepancies. The main discrepancy is that it will rarely be known whether the two groups under comparison are identical in various characteristics, especially with regard to the nature and severity of the disease. Besides, certain diseases will have a tendency to change over a period of time with regard to severity. This may be either due to natural causes or may be due to vast preventive measures undertaken or may be due to changes in living habits. Hence either mild or severe cases of the disease may be more prevalent at one time of investigation as compared to the other. The result of the treatment of milder cases cannot be compared with the results of the treatment of severe cases or vice-versa. Similarly the method of diagnosis of the cases by different workers will also influence the type of cases, severity of the disease, etc. Besides, the reaction of patients to various drugs under different conditions will not be the same. Keeping all these factors in view, it will not be valid to compare the results of one experiment with the results of another conducted in the past, unless it can be wholly taken as that the two groups are identical in all respects referred to above, which may rarely exist.

b. Patient as his Own Control

All patients will not react equally to any drug. This variability amongst different patients to the drug can be overcome by recording the results on the same patient before and after treatment in certain types of experiments. In such cases, a group of patients is selected and the observations on desired characteristics are recorded before treatment for each of the patient. After administering the treatment to the group the results are again recorded and the comparisons are made between the 'initial' and 'after treatment' values. In this case the patients serve as their own controls. In using such a control, the basic assumption will be that the patient will not have variations over a period of time with regard to response to the drug, severity of the symptom and also that there is no carry over effect from any treatment which the patient might have had previously. Validity of such assumptions can be established by conducting preliminary investigations on small groups, which are known as pilot investigations.

Diagrammatically this can be represented as follows:

Measurement before treatment (X)	Treatment Introduced	Measurement after treatment (Y)

Treatment effect = (X) – (Y)

c. Concurrent Control

For human beings, in many cases the initial effect cannot be estimated or for animals the results to be compared between various treatments cannot be obtained without sacrificing the animal under experimentation. Hence in such cases the different treatments are administered to different identical groups. Out of these groups all may receive different treatments between which comparisons are made or one group is kept as a control group receiving only a placebo or a previously known drug against which the other groups are compared.

The measurements may be made only at the end of the trail on all the groups where such measurements are known as *'After only with control'*. Here the effect of treatment is assessed as the difference in measurements between the groups.

Group I	Treatment administered	Measurement after treatment (Y)
Group II	Placebo or some other treatment	Measurement after treatment (Z)
	Treatment effect = (Y) – (Z)	

Here the assumption is that all the treatment groups are identical at the start of experimentation.

If the above assumption is not valid, measurements have to be made both at the start of experimentation as well as at the end. Effect of the treatment is assessed as difference between the change in the initial and after treatment values individually in the control and experimental groups. Such a comparison is known as *'Before and after with control'*.

Group I	Measurement before treatment (X)	Treatment administered	Measurement made after treatment (Y)
Group I	Measurement before treatment (A)	Treatment administered or Placebo	Measurement made after treatment (Z)

Treatment effect = (Y – X) - (Z – A)

Formal Designs for Clinical Trials

There are various formal designs used in clinical trials. Some of them are illustrated below:

I. *Completely Randomised Design*

i. Involves principle of randomisation and replication.
ii. Treatments are assigned to experimental units at random.
iii. If ten subjects are there, two treatments are allocated at random to the patients. Five get treatment A and another five get treatment B.
iv. Used when experimental units are homogeneously distributed.

II. *Randomised Block Design*

i. Principle of randomisation and local control is ensured in this design.
ii. All the units in the sample are divided into certain number of homogeneous groups according to the number of treatments to be administered.
iii. All the units in a particular group are allocated a particular treatment at random. Thus the treatment is allocated on group basis and not on individual patient basis as was done in the case of Completely Randomised Design.
iv. In this design number of treatments would be equal to the number of groups of patients.

Diagrammatically the design is represented below.

Treatments	Group of patients
I	Group 1
II	Group 2
III	Group 3
IV	Group 4

III. *Latin Square Design*

i. Experimental units are arranged into certain number of groups equal to the number of treatments.
ii. Each group is again divided into certain number of subgroups equal to the number of treatments.
iii. They are arranged into rows and columns as shown in the diagram below.
iv. Each treatment is allocated to these subgroups such that it appears once in each row and column.
v. This design enables elimination of variability across units and treatment effects.

If there are four grades of the disease status, the patients of these grades are arranged into rows and columns as shown in the diagram and four treatments A, B, C, D are allocated to each group of patients as shown in the diagram, so that each treatment appears only once in each row and column.

Variations in disease status

Grade 1	Grade 2	Grade 3	Grade 4
A	B	C	D
B	C	D	A
C	D	A	B
D	A	B	C

IV. *Factorial Designs*

In a simple experimental design, if there are three drugs each with three doses, the effect of different drugs along with different doses can be studied by administering the drugs and doses independently. But this design yields only the effect of different drugs and doses independently, but not the effect of combination of drugs and doses. But if it is desired to know the interaction between the drugs and doses, Factorial designs are to be used.

In Factorial designs it is possible to assess the effect of various factors such as main treatments, effect of doses of treatment, effect of treatment and doses on different stages of disease, interaction between the main treatment and the doses of treatment, interaction between doses of treatment and stages of disease and the interaction between main treatment, doses of treatment and stages of disease.

The factorial designs may be simple or complex as illustrated in the following diagrams.

In these diagrams each box represents a group of patients treated with particular drug and dose or regimen of treatment.

Simple factorial design is suitable if the effect of only drug and doses of drugs are to be studied as illustrated below, where each box represents one block of patients.

Simple factorial design

Drug 1 & Dose 1	Drug 1 & Dose 2	Drug 1 & Dose 3
Drug 2 & Dose 1	Drug 2 & Dose 2	Drug 2 & Dose 3
Drug 3 & Dose 1	Drug 3 & Dose 2	Drug 3 & Dose 3

When the effect of different drugs, doses of drugs as well as regimen of drugs are to be studied a complex factorial design can be adopted as illustrated below, where each box represents one block of patients.

Complex factorial design

Drug 1, Dose 1 Regimen 1	Drug 1, Dose 2 Regimen 1	Drug 1, Dose 3 Regimen 1
Drug 1, Dose 1 Regimen 2	Drug 1, Dose 2 Regimen 2	Drug 1, Dose 3 Regimen 2
Drug 2, Dose 1 Regimen 1	Drug 2, Dose 2 Regimen 1	Drug 2, Dose 3 Regimen 1

Drug 2, Dose 1 Regimen 2	Drug 2, Dose 2 Regimen 2	Drug 2, Dose 3 Regimen 2
Drug 3, Dose 1 Regimen 1	Drug 3, Dose 2 Regimen 1	Drug 3, Dose 3 Regimen 1
Drug 3, Dose 1 Regimen 2	Drug 3, Dose 2 Regimen 2	Drug 3, Dose 3 Regimen 2

No. of subjects or experimental units may be same or different in each block of the design. If the numbers are same it facilitates analysis.

Analysis can be carried out to answer questions such as:

a. Whether different drugs influence the outcome?
b. Whether different doses of drugs affect the outcome ?
c. Whether regimens of drugs affect the outcome ?
d. Is there any interaction between the dose and type of drug?
e. Is there any interaction between the regimen and type of drug ?
f. Is there any interaction between the regimen and dose of drug ?
g. Is there any interaction between the type, regimen and dose of drug ?

V. *Crossover Designs*

In order to eliminate 'between group variations', a design, which can be adopted, is a *Crossover design*. In this design the variation is only 'within subjects' rather than 'between subjects'. In this type of design the same group of patients are given both the treatments of interest in sequence. The second treatment is applied to patients, after neutralisation of carry over effect of the previous treatment. A wash out period may have to be introduced after the first treatment is administered. In this design the disadvantage may be that the patients may drop out after first treatment and may not be available to receive the second treatment. This design may not be suitable if the first drug cures the disease or the drug is effective only during a particular stage of the disease or if the disease status changes radically during the period of study.

VI. *Sequential Trials*

Ethically a patient should not be treated by an inferior drug or for a prolonged duration. To take care of these factors, it may be preferable to set up a *'Sequential trial'* where the sample size is determined during the course of the trial. In this design the outcome is studied after each case is treated with the drug and the study is terminated when once the outcome reaches a desired criteria. In this design the decision lines or control charts of continuing or terminating the trial are drawn at the start of the trial on some predetermined criteria through statistical procedures. This is equivalent to the quality control techniques applied in industries, where a certain batch of products are either accepted or rejected for quality on some pre-determined criteria. The advantage of this design is that the number of patients required for the study would be less than the other designs. However sequential trials are inappropriate if the duration of outcome is long.

Blinding During Trials

Errors may occur during assessment of results due to the bias of experimenter, if he knows what treatment is administered to a particular group. Treatment effect may also be different if the patient knows what treatment has been administered to him/her. Even the person analysing the results may be influenced by the treatment schedule to the patients. To overcome these errors usually blinding of treatments is done.

Blinding can be done by not informing the patient as to what treatment has been administered. This type of blinding is known as *Single blind trial*. In order to avoid experimenter's bias, both the experimenter as well as the patient is kept unaware of the treatment schedule. This type of blinding is known as *Double blind trial*. If the person analysing the results of the experiment is also kept unaware of the treatment schedule then it is known as *Triple blind trial*.

Sample Size

The trial should be conducted on an adequate sample size, which would detect reliably the small or moderate but clinically important differences between the treatment groups.

In clinical trials usually there will be two groups, one experimental and the other control group. In order to estimate the size of sample for each group, the difference in the response rates as well as the variability in the response rates of the two groups are to be taken into consideration and the sample size is estimated from the following formula.

$$n = [(p_1q_1 + p_2q_2) (z_\alpha + z_\beta)^2] / (p_1 - p_2)^2$$

n is the adequate sample size for each group

p_1 is the expected response in the treatment group and p_2 in the control group

and $q_1 = (1 - p_1)$ $q_2 = (1 - p_2)$

z_α is the value of the Standard normal variate corresponding to a significance level of α (usually taken as 1.96 for a two tailed test at 0.05 level).

z_β is the value of the Standard normal variate corresponding to the desired level of power of the test (usually taken as 1.24 for a power of 80%).

The values for p_1 and p_2 are usually obtained from pilot studies or assumptions from some other studies.

Example 11.1. If an investigator wants to estimate the cure rate amongst anaemia cases by administration of particular drug compared against a known drug, minimum number of cases in each group to be investigated is calculated as follows:

Suppose, from pilot study it is known that the response rate in the new drug is 80% and the previously known drug was 40%, then the sample size is estimated as follows:

p_1 the expected response in the new treatment group = 80% or 0.80

p_2 the expected response in the previously known drug = 40% or 0.40

$q_1 = (1 - 0.80) = 0.20$

$q_2 = (1 - 0.40) = 0.60$

z_α is the value of the standard normal variate corresponding to a significance level of 0.05 taken as 1.96.

z_β is the value of the standard normal variate corresponding to the desired level of power of the test, taken as 1.24 for a power of 80% .

$$n = [(p_1q_1 + p_2q_2)(z_\alpha + z_\beta)^2] / (p_1 - p_2)^2$$

$$= \frac{[(0.80 \times 0.20) + (0.40 \text{ X } 0.60)]\,(1.96 + 1.24)^2}{(0.80 - 0.40)^2}$$

$$= \frac{[(0.16) + (0.24)]\ (10.24)}{(0.40)^2}$$

$$= \frac{(0.40)\ (10.24)}{(0.16)}$$

$$= (4.096) / (0.16)$$

= 26 cases are required to be investigated in each group.

Chapter 12 Sampling Variation and Tests of Significance

Sampling Variation

Most of the biological investigations are carried out on samples as it will not be possible to cover the entire population. It is known that repeated samples even though from the same population will not yield the same estimates for any characteristic under observation. As an example, if four samples of 25 persons from a common population are considered and the mean pulse rate of persons in these samples are calculated, then it will be seen that all these four means will not be exactly equal. This is because there is always variability amongst observations and this variability is common amongst biological observations.

Such a difference between the sample estimates, even though the samples are from the same population, is known as the *Sampling variation*. Whenever two or more samples are considered, the differences observed in the sample estimates of a particular characteristic may be either due to sampling variation or may be due to the fact that the samples might have come from different populations with different values for the characteristic.

As such, whenever dealing with the estimates from two or more samples or groups one would be interested to know whether the differences observed for the value of the estimates between the groups are only due to the sampling variation or otherwise. In other words, one would be interested to know whether the samples are coming from the same population or different populations. For sorting out this, one should know the range of the estimate, which a characteristic can take if different samples are taken from the same population. This range depends upon the mean value, the variability of the observations in the original population and also on the size of the sample.

The methodologies of statistics which deal with the techniques to analyse, how far the differences between the estimates from different samples are due to sampling variation or otherwise is known as the *Testing of hypothesis*. In this methodology, the probability, that the difference between the sample estimates attributable to the sampling variation is worked out by several methods.

Some Terms Used in Tests of Significance

Before discussing the details of testing of hypothesis it is necessary to understand the meaning of some of the terms used in procedures of testing of hypothesis.

i. *Null Hypothesis*

The first step in the testing of hypothesis is to set up a hypothesis appropriate with the problem and this hypothesis is usually in the form of a null hypothesis. The null hypothesis should be framed in such a way that it conveys the meaning that the difference between the estimates provided by different samples is due to sampling variation. In other words, the null hypothesis states that the samples are coming out of a common population.

Going back to the example of pulse rates of persons given earlier, the appropriate null hypothesis which may be stated is that the mean pulse rates of all the four groups are same or in other words all the four samples are from a population with a common mean.

In clinical medicine, an experiment may be carried out to test the effectiveness of a new drug over a standard drug. There may be two groups of patients, each group being treated with a particular drug. Suppose the effectiveness of the drug is measured by the proportion of patients who are cured in each group, then the appropriate null hypothesis in this experiment would be that the proportion of patients cured in the new treatment group may be same as that of the proportion of patients cured in the standard treatment group.

ii. *Level of Significance*

Having framed a null hypothesis, that the two groups are from the same population, it is necessary to fix the magnitude of the risk of making a wrong conclusion of rejecting the null hypothesis. This quantity is calculated in terms of a probability level denoted by P and is called as the level of significance. P gives the probability of the sampling variation or the chance factor being responsible for the causation of the difference in the estimates of the samples, when the samples are from the same population. In other words, this gives the probability level to decide whether the null hypothesis is to be rejected or not. If the value of P is small, it means that the probability of attributing the difference between sample estimates to the sampling variation or chance factor is small. On the other hand, if P is large then the probability that the difference between the sample estimates caused by sampling variation is large. As such, whenever P is small the null hypothesis is rejected. Incidentally it may be noted that the value of P also gives the size of the risk factor in making a wrong conclusion. While accepting or rejecting the null hypothesis one may commit two types of errors. If the null hypothesis is rejected when it is actually true, one will have committed a *Type I error*. On the contrary, if null hypothesis is accepted when it is false, *Type II error* is committed.

How small should be this value of P to reject a null hypothesis depends upon the type of investigation. One should be careful in deciding the size of P. A balance between Type I error and Type II error is to be made, depending upon the gravity of making such errors in the conclusions to be made from the study. As a matter of practical convenience a value of less than or equal to 0.05 is the usual level which is commonly accepted for rejecting the null hypothesis. By this it means that one would be going wrong in 5 out of 100 cases by rejecting the null hypothesis. Smaller the value of P, it is more evident that the differences between the estimates of the samples are significant. All tests of significance are aimed at finding this value of P.

iii. *Standard Error*

It is the standard deviation of a statistical parameter like mean, proportion, etc. This gives an idea about the dispersion of the above statistical parameters obtained from repeated samples from the same population.

In other words, the standard error of a mean is the standard deviation of all means of several samples taken from the same population. Similarly, standard error of a proportion is the standard deviation of proportions of several samples of a qualitative data taken from the same population.

Standard error can be estimated from a single sample and the standard errors of mean and proportion are given by the following expressions.

$$\text{Standard error of mean} = s/(\sqrt{n})$$

Where s is the standard deviation of observations in the observed sample and n is the number of observations in the sample.

$$\text{Standard error of a proportion} = \sqrt{(pq/n)}$$

where p is the proportion of occurrence of an event in the observed sample, $q = (1-p)$ and n is the number of observations in the sample.

Standard error is useful for fixing the *Confidence limits,* which gives a range for the statistical parameter, indicating that the true value of the parameter is contained in the range with a certain confidence. In other words a 95% confidence interval of mean gives a range which indicates the true value of the mean is within the range with 95% confidence, or in other words, 95% of the sample estimates will lie within this range.

Standard error is basic statistical quantity for testing the significance of the difference in estimates between two samples.

General Procedure for Testing of a Hypothesis

The following are the steps involved in applying a test of significance:

i) Set up a null hypothesis suitable to the problem either in qualitative or quantitative terms.
ii) Define the alternate hypothesis, if necessary
iii) Calculate the suitable test statistics, t, χ^2, F, etc. using the relevant formula.
iv) Determine the degrees of freedom for the test statistics.
v) Find out the probability level, P corresponding to the calculated value of the test statistics and its degrees of freedom. This can be read from the relevant tables. This gives the probability that the difference between the sample estimates is because of sampling variation.
iv) Generally, reject the null hypothesis, if P is less than or equal to 0.05, otherwise accept it. In other words the difference between the two sample estimates is considered as significant if P is less than or equal to 0.05.

Conclusions are usually made on the basis of tests of significance that the two samples are from the same population or not without considering the direction of the difference between the two sample estimates like mean or proportion. Such tests are known as *two tailed tests*. On the other hand if conclusions are to be made as to whether one of the sample mean is larger than the other, tests of significance in such cases are known as *one tailed test*. In one tailed test the table value of P is taken as half the tabulated value.

Test for Large Samples

i. *To test the Difference between Two Means or Proportions*

A sample is usually considered to be large if the number of observations is more than 30. In such samples, the estimate may be either in terms of qualitative data or quantitative data. Depending upon the nature of data, appropriate tests are to be applied.

Generally the biological observations on large samples are distributed as a Normal distribution. However, all means or proportions from large samples follow a Normal distribution. Similarly the difference between two means or proportions are also distributed as a Normal distribution, with mean zero and a standard deviation equal to the standard error of the difference between the two sample estimates. This standard error is computed from the respective standard errors of the parameters under comparison.

The standard error of the difference between the two means or proportion is equal to

$$\sqrt{\{(SE_1)^2 + (SE_2)^2\}}$$

where (SE_1) and (SE_2) are the standard errors, which is estimated for mean equal to $(s/\sqrt{n})$ and for a proportion equal to $\sqrt{(pq/n)}$.

The standard error of the difference between the two sample means is:

$$\sqrt{\{(s_1^2/n_1) + (s_2^2/n_2)\}}$$

where s_1 and s_2 are the standard deviations of the two samples and n_1 and n_2 are their sample sizes respectively.

The standard error of the difference between the two proportions is given by the expression,

$$\sqrt{\{(p_1 q_1/n_1) + (p_2 q_2/n_2)\}}$$

where p_1 and p_2 are the estimates of the proportions of the event in the two samples and q_1 and q_2 are equal to $(1-p_1)$ and $(1-p_2)$ respectively n_1 and n_2 are the number of observations in the two samples.

It was mentioned that the difference between the sample means or proportions follow a Normal distribution with mean zero and standard deviation equal to the standard error of the difference.

Hence it is possible to find the probability whether the difference between the two sample estimates is due to sampling variation or not. This probability level is given in the Normal distribution tables (Appendix Table 5) corresponding to the ratio of the difference between the means or proportions and the standard error of this difference.

The following procedure is adopted for testing for the significance of the difference between means or proportions.

i) Calculate the two means $\overline{x}_1$ and $\overline{x}_2$ or proportion p_1 and p_2 corresponding to the two samples with sample size n_1 and n_2 respectively.
ii) Set up the null hypothesis that the two samples are from the same population and that the difference between the two sample estimates is due to sampling variation.
iii) Calculate the standard deviation of the two samples and their standard errors (SE_1) and (SE_2) respectively.
iv) Calculate the standard error of the difference between the two sample estimates as

$$\sqrt{\{(SE_1)^2 + (SE_2)^2\}}$$

v) Calculate the quantity critical ratio (CR) or z value z = (Difference between sample estimates / SE of difference)
vi) Refer to the Normal distribution table and corresponding to this calculated value of z, find the value of probability P.
vii) If P is less than or equal to 0.05, reject the null hypothesis and conclude that the difference between the two sample estimates as significant.

If P is greater than 0.05 accept the null hypothesis and conclude that the difference between the two sample estimates as not significant.

Example 12.1. In an epidemic of gastroenteritis in an area the number of cases reported in two populations consuming water from different sources were as follows:

Source of water	No. of people consuming water from the source	No. of cases of gastroenteritis
Tap water	800	35
Hand pump	2400	120
Total	**3200**	**155**

From the above data it is desired to find out whether the difference in the proportion of cases in the two groups is significantly different.

i) The null hypothesis in this case is that the difference is not significant.

ii) p_1 = Proportion of cases amongst tap water consumers
= (35 / 800)
= 0.044
$q_1 = (1 - p_1) = (1 - 0.044) = 0.956$
n_1 = no. of tap water consumers = 800

iii) Standard error of the proportion p_1, (SE_1)
$= \sqrt{(p_1 q_1 / n_1)}$
$= \sqrt{\{(0.044 \times 0.956) / 800\}}$
$= \sqrt{(0.0000525)} = 0.0072$

iv) p_2 = Proportion of cases amongst hand pump water consumers
= (120/2400) = 0.05
$q_2 = (1 - p_2)$
$= (1 - 0.05) = 0.95$
n_2 = No. of hand pump water consumers = 2400

v) Standard error of the proportion p_2, (SE_2)
$= \sqrt{(p_2 q_2 / n_2)}$
$= \sqrt{\{(0.05 \times 0.95) / 2400\}}$
$= \sqrt{(0.0000198)} = 0.0044$

vi) Difference between the proportions = (0.050 – 0.044)
= 0.006

vii) Standard error of this difference $= \sqrt{\{(SE_1)^2 + (SE_2)^2\}}$
$= \sqrt{(0.0000525 + 0.0000197)}$
$= \sqrt{(0.0000722)} = 0.0085$

vi) Z or CR of Difference between the proportions
= (0.006/0.0085)
= 0.706

ix) From Normal distribution table, (Appendix 5)
P corresponding to this value of Z is more than 0.48

This means that the probability, that sampling variation is the cause of the difference in the proportion of cases between the two groups is more than 0.48.

Hence the null hypothesis is not rejected and it is concluded that the difference is not statistically significant.

Tests for Comparing Means of Small Samples

In the methods used for testing of large samples using Normal distribution, the standard errors were estimated from the sample standard deviations. This estimate should be consistent from sample to sample. But this is a statistical parameter subject to sampling variations. With small samples these variations will be large and the estimate of standard error will be inconsistent from sample to sample and as such it will not be accurate. The Normal probability calculated using this inconsistent estimate will not be correct. Hence in 1908, 'Student' derived a new distribution, known as 't' distribution. Tables have been constructed giving the probability levels of several values of this statistics t (Appendix Table 3). The value of t is dependent upon the sample size 'n' and for each value of the degrees of freedom used for estimating the standard deviation of the sample, the value of t is different. Hence the table of t-values covers the various degrees of freedom and gives the probability levels for the calculated values of t at each degrees of freedom.

In actual working, the t-statistics is calculated as a ratio of the difference between the two means to the standard error of the difference between the means.

$$t = (\bar{x}_1 - \bar{x}_2) / S_{md}$$

where, $\bar{x}_1$ and $\bar{x}_2$ are the means of the two samples and S_{md} is the standard error of the difference between the means.

In actual experiments, the observations may be carried out on two independent samples, one known as the control group and the other known as the treated group. The means of these two groups may be compared for their significant difference.

In such cases the comparisons are said to be unpaired comparisons. In some other experiments to overcome the variability between the groups, the observations may be carried out on a single sample and the values of a certain characteristic may be noted before and after the treatment with any particular drug. In such cases, the comparisons of values of observations are known as paired comparisons.

The method of estimating the standard error and S_{md} is slightly different in the two cases and they are detailed below.

a) *t-test for comparing paired observations*

The formula for the calculation of t-statistics in this case being

$$t = (\bar{d} / s_{md}) \text{ with } (n - 1) \text{ d.f.}$$

where, ($\bar{d}$ is the mean of the differences in the values of the variable of the sample observations before and after treatment and n is the number of observations in the sample.

s_{md} is the standard error of the mean difference and is calculated by the formula:

$$s_{md} = (s_d / \sqrt{n})$$

where, s_d is the standard deviation of the values of d, the differences in the variable before and after the treatment.

The steps in the calculation of t-test for paired observations are as follows:-

i) Calculate the difference d_i for each pair of observations before and after treatment and compute their mean $\bar{d}$

ii) Set up the null hypothesis that $\bar{d} = 0$

iii) Calculate the standard deviation of these differences s_d

$$= \frac{\sqrt{[\Sigma(\text{Difference between individual observation and } \bar{d})^2]}}{(n-1)}$$

Where n is the number of pairs of observations

iv) Calculate the standard error s_{md} from the formula

$$s_{md} = (s_d / \sqrt{n})$$

v) Calculate the value of t-statistics as $t = (\bar{d} / s_{md})$

vi) Compute the degrees of freedom as (n – 1).

vii) From the t-distribution table, (Appendix 3) find the probability level corresponding to this value of t and degrees of freedom (n –1).

viii) If $P < 0.05$ reject the null hypothesis and conclude that the difference between before and after treatment values are significant.

Example 12.2. On a group of anaemic patients, an iron preparation was administered and the haemoglobin levels of the patients before and after therapy were noted and are given below. It is desired to find out whether there is a significant change in the haemoglobin level of the group after the therapy. The steps for the calculation are worked out below:

Patient No.	Hb. level in gm%		Difference between after & before therapy (d)	$(d - \bar{d})$	$(d - \bar{d})^2$
	Before therapy	After therapy			
1	5.6	10.2	4.6	1.87	3.50
2	4.8	9.4	4.6	1.87	3.50
3	6.5	11.0	4.5	1.77	3.13
4	7.5	7.5	0.0	–2.73	7.45
5	4.5	7.5	3.0	–0.27	0.07
6	3.5	6.0	2.5	–0.23	0.05
7	6.7	8.0	1.3	–1.43	2.04
8	6.2	9.6	3.4	0.67	0.45
9	5.6	10.0	4.4	1.67	2.79
10	4.4	8.4	4.0	1.27	1.61
11	7.5	8.0	0.5	–2.23	4.97
12	8.0	8.0	0.0	–2.73	7.45
Total			**32.8**		**37.01**

i) Null hypothesis is that there is no significant change due to therapy.

ii) Mean differences in Hb level before and after therapy,

$$\bar{d} = (32.8/12) = 2.73 \approx 2.7$$

iii) Standard deviation of the differences $= \sqrt{(37.01/11)}$

$$= 1.834$$

iv) Standard error of the mean difference = $(1.834/\sqrt{12})$
$= (1.834/3.464)$
$= 0.530$

v) $t = \dfrac{\text{(Mean difference in Hb. before \& after therapy)}}{\text{SE of mean difference}}$

$= (2.73/0.530) = 5.15$

From t-tables, corresponding to 11 d.f. and the calculated value of t = 5.15 , P< 0.001.

This means that the null hypothesis is rejected and it is concluded that the mean difference is statistically significant.

b) *t-test for comparing the means of two independent samples*

For comparing means of two independent samples, t-test statistics is calculated from the formula:

$$t = \{ (\bar{x}_1 - \bar{x}_2)/S_{md} \}$$

Here S_{md} is the estimated standard error of the difference between the two sample means and is obtained as follows:

$$s_{md} = \sqrt{[\{(n_1 + n_2)/n_1 n_2\}\{(n_1 - 1) s_1^2 + (n_2 - 1) s_2^2)\}/(n_1 + n_2 - 2)]}$$

Where s_1^2 and s_2^2 are the standard deviations of the two samples and n_1 and n_2 are their respective sample sizes. Thus

$$t = \frac{\bar{x}_1 - \bar{x}_2}{\sqrt{[\{(n_1 + n_2)/n_1 n_2\}\{(n_1 - 1) s_1^2 + (n_2 - 1)s_2^2)\}/(n_1 + n_2 - 2)]}}$$

with $(n_1 + n_2 - 2)$ df

Example 12.3. In an experiment to know whether there is any difference in the length of small intestines between males and females, the observations recorded were as follows:

	Males	Females
No. of observations	17	15
Mean length of the small intestines	157"	146"
SD of the observations	34"	31"

To find out whether there is any significant difference between the length of small intestines between the two sex groups, t-test can be applied and interpreted as follows:

First a null hypothesis is formulated that the difference between the means is due to sampling variation.

Then t - is calculated from the above formula.

Here

$\bar{x}_1$	=	157"	$\bar{x}_2$	=	146"
s_1	=	34"	s_2	=	31"
n_1	=	17	n_2	=	15

Substituting the above values in the formula:

$$t = \frac{(157 - 146)}{\sqrt{[\{(17+15) / 17 \times 15\} \{16 (34)^2 + 14(31)^2\} / (17 + 15 - 2)]}}$$

$= (11) / \sqrt{[\{(32/255) (31950/30)\}]}$

$= (11) / \sqrt{(133.5)}$

$= (11) / (11.56) = 0.95$

The above t value has $(n_1 + n_2 - 2) = 30$ df

Referring to the table of t-distribution at 30 d.f., it is seen that the calculated value lies between 0.854 and 1.055 with corresponding P values between 0.40, and 0.30. That is to say that $0.40 > P > 0.30$. This indicates that the difference between the two sample means can be attributed to sampling variation with a probability more than 0.30.

As seen earlier the value of P to consider a difference as significant, should be less than 0.05.

Hence the null hypothesis is accepted and the difference in the mean length of small intestines between the two sexes is taken as not significant.

To test for an alternative hypothesis that $\bar{x}_1$ is greater than or less than $(\bar{x}_2)$, *one tailed test* is used where, half the probability level located from the t-table is used.

In the present example, if we want to test whether the mean length of male intestine is more than the mean length of female intestine, half of the P value located from the table, equivalent to $P > 0.15$ is considered, which still allows us to accept the null hypotheses that the length of small intestines amongst males is not longer than those of females.

The usual assumptions underlying the t-distribution is that the means of the two samples are normally and independently distributed and that the variances of the two samples are equal. This equality of variances can be tested by F-test, which is the ratio of the variances of the two samples. However, even when the variance of the two samples turn out to be unequal, still the t-test is applicable with a correction for significance level suggested by Cochran. This method satisfies most of the practical situations.

By this method, t is calculated from the usual formula and the significance level of this calculated t is noted for $(n_1 - 1)$ and $(n_2 - 1)$ d.f., where n_1 and n_2 are the two sample sizes. If these two probabilities are termed as P_1 and P_2, the actual significance level of the calculated t is obtained as the weighted average of P_1 and P_2 in relation to their respective squares of standard errors:

i.e. $P = (w_1P_1 + w_2P_2) / (w_1 + w_2)$

Where w_1 and w_2 are the squares of the standard errors of the two sample means.

χ^2 Test for Qualitative Data

a. *χ^2 Test for $r \times c$ table*

In the previous sections it was seen that when the data is measured in quantitative measurements the difference between the two sample means can be tested by t-test. However, when the data is measured in terms of attributes, it is essential to test whether the differences in the distribution of attributes in different samples are due to sampling variation or otherwise. As an example if there are two groups, one consisting of healthy individuals and another with a particular disease, say different types of leprosy, and if it is desired to elicit whether the blood group distribution has any association with the incidence of the disease, then the blood group distribution amongst healthy individuals is to be compared with the diseased group and any difference between the two groups in this regard is to be tested for significance. In such cases χ^2 (chi-square) test is applied.

In calculating χ^2 test statistics, an estimate of the expected number of frequencies for each blood group, both for the healthy group and the diseased group is calculated under the null hypothesis and χ^2 is obtained as :

$$\chi^2 = \Sigma \{(\text{Observed frequency} - \text{Expected frequency})^2 / \text{Expected frequency}\}$$

The above value is calculated for each of the cell in the table and sum of the above ratios is the total chi-square value.

As in t-test, χ^2 statistics also depends upon the degrees of freedom. Hence the calculated χ^2 is referred for its significance level, P, from the χ^2 distribution table (Appendix table 4) corresponding to its degrees of freedom. The degrees of freedom is obtained as the product of (c-1) and (r-1) where c is the number of columns, i.e. the number of groups compared and r is the number of rows, i.e. number of alternatives in each group.

As in the case of t-test, if P is more than 0.05 the difference between the groups is attributed to sampling variation and is considered as not significant and the null hypothesis is accepted and thus concluded that there may not be any association between the attributes and the groups. If P is less than 0.05, the conclusion would be otherwise.

As an illustration, in the example 12.4 of incidence of leprosy, P obtained from the calculated χ^2 is less than 0.05, and hence the probability that the sampling variation is the cause for the difference in the blood group distribution between healthy and leprosy groups is less than 0.05 and hence the conclusion would be that the blood group distributions of healthy and leprosy groups may be different. From the data further investigations have to be made to find out as to which of the blood groups are more differing between the two groups.

Example 12.4. The data given in the following table gives distribution of non-leprosy, lepromatous leprosy and non-lepromatous leprosy cases according to the blood group of the persons.

Blood group	Non-leprosy	Lepromatous leprosy	Non-lepromatous leprosy	Total
A	30	49	52	131
B	60	49	36	145
O	47	59	48	154
AB	13	12	16	41
Total	**150**	**169**	**152**	**471**

To understand whether the blood group is associated with the incidence of leprosy, χ^2 test is applied as follows.

First the null hypothesis is formulated that the blood group distributions are same in all the three groups.

For calculating χ^2, the expected frequencies for each cell is obtained with the assumption that the blood group distribution of each of the sub group would be same as that of total series. That is to say, that for each of the groups of non leprosy, lepromatous leprosy and non-lepromatous leprosy, the total frequency of each of the groups, i.e. 150, 169 and 152 is distributed into A, B, O and AB groups in the ratio of (131: 145 : 154 : 41) which corresponds to the ratio of blood group distribution of the entire series.

Thus, *expected frequency* for each cell is calculated as follows:.

Blood group	Non-leprosy	Lepromatous leprosy	Non-lepromatous leprosy
A	(131/471) x 150 = 41.7	(131/471) x 169 = 47.0	(131/471) x 152 =42.3
B	(145/471) x 150 = 46.2	(145/471) x 169 = 52.0	(145/471) x 152 =46.8
C	(154/471) x 150 = 49.0	(154/471) x 169 = 55.3	(154/471) x 152 =49.7
AB	(41/471) x 150 = 13.1	(41/471) x 169 = 14.7	(41/471) x 152 =13.2

Then χ^2 is obtained as $\{(O-E)^2/E\}$ for each cell where O and E corresponds to observed and expected frequencies for the corresponding cells.

χ^2 value for each cell is as follows:

Blood group	Non-leprosy	Lepromatous leprosy	Non-lepromatous leprosy	Total
A	3.28	0.09	2.22	5.59
B	4.12	0.17	2.49	6.78
O	0.08	0.25	0.06	0.39
AB	0.00	0.50	0.59	1.09
Total	**7.48**	**1.01**	**5.36**	**13.85**

The sum of χ^2 for all the cells = 13.85

The degree of freedom for the above table

= (3 – 1) x (4–1) = 2 x 3 = 6

From χ^2 distribution tables P for this calculated χ^2 at 6 df is between 0.02 and 0.05 which less than 0.05.

This means that the probability of sampling variation being the cause of differences in the blood group distribution of different groups is less than 0.05.

The null hypothesis is rejected and concluded that the differences in the blood group distributions of the three groups are significant.

In order to understand which of the blood groups are more prone to leprosy, the contribution to the total χ^2 from each of the cells is to be examined. From the table it is seen that the maximum contributions are from B and A groups.

Further tests applicable to proportions can be applied to test the differences between the portion of A and non-A or B and non-B groups for cells which have contributed maximum χ^2, and conclusions can be made to ascertain the association of these particular blood groups with the incidence of leprosy.

b. *χ^2 Test for 2 × 2 table*

The exact method of calculating χ^2 in the case of 2 x 2 table where the number of rows and columns are exactly two is simple. As an example, if a sample of population is classified according to their sex as well as those with a particular disease or no disease within each sex, it may be necessary to find out whether the proportion of the diseased in each sex is same or not. In other words it has to be tested whether the difference observed between the two sexes in the prevalence of the disease is due to sampling variation or otherwise.

In such cases χ^2 is calculated as illustrated further.

The data can be tabulated as follows:

Disease status	Male	Female	Total
With disease	a	b	**(a+b)**
Without disease	c	d	**(c+d)**
Total	**(a+c)**	**(b+d)**	**G**

where a, b, c and d are the frequencies in the respective cells and G is equal to (a + b + c + d), the total sample size.

$$\chi^2 = \frac{(ad - bc)^2 \text{ x } G}{(a+b)\ (c+d)\ (a+c)\ (b+d)}$$

The degrees of freedom for the above χ^2 is 1, since

(c–1) x (r–1) = 1 where c = r = 2

When the expected frequency in any cell is less than 5, a correction suggested by Yates is to be applied for the calculation of χ^2. This correction is also known as correction for continuity.

After applying Yates correction,

$$\chi^2 = \frac{[\,|\ (ad-bc)\ | - G/2]^2 \text{ x } G}{(a+b)\ (c+d)\ (a+c)\ (b+d)}$$

Example 12.5. In a Filariasis survey, the number of people with and without filariasis infestation in the two sex groups were as follows. In order to find out whether the prevalence of filariasis has any association with the sex, χ^2 test is applied as follows.

Filariasis infestation	Male	Female	Total
Yes	28	20	48
No	237	222	459
Total	**265**	**242**	**507**

The first step is to set up a null hypothesis, that the difference in the filariasis prevalence in the two sex groups is due to sampling variation.

χ^2 is calculated by substituting the above values in the formula as follows:

$$\chi^2 = \frac{[(28 \times 222) - (20 \times 237)]^2 \times 507}{265 \times 242 \times 48 \times 459}$$

$= 0.78$

P value corresponding to this value of χ^2 at 1 df is more than 0.30.

This means that the probability that the difference in the prevalence rates of filariasis infestation between the two sexes which can be attributed to the sampling variation is more than 0.30.

As such the null hypothesis is accepted and concluded that the difference is not significant.

In the above example, Yates correction is not applied as the frequencies in each cell is sufficiently large.

c. *Fisher's exact probability test for 2 × 2 tables*

Chi-square test in 2 x 2 table relies on a large sample approximation and in situations where a large sample assumption is not valid, Chi-square test of independence provides only approximate results. In such situations where a large sample assumption is not valid, Fisher's exact test provides exact one-tailed and two-tailed P-values for a given frequency table. Fisher's exact test computes the probability for occurrence of exactly the same frequencies as observed in each cell under null hypothesis. If the Probability is less than 0.05, the null hypothesis is rejected.

As given in the above example if, a, b, c and d are the frequencies in the four cells of 2 x 2 table (a + c), (b + d) are the column totals and (a + b), (c + d) are the row totals, then the probability of observing the respective number of observation in each cell is given by:

$$P = [\{(a + c)!\ (b + d)!\ (a + b)!\ (c + d)!\} \ / \ \{ n!\ a!\ b!\ c!\ d! \}]$$

Where n is the total number of observations and (!) sign refers to factorial.

Example 12.6. If the number of boys and girls who are regular in their exercises is distributed as given below, it is required to test whether there is any significant difference in the exercise habits between boys and girls.

Habit	Boys	Girls	Total
Exercise regularly	2	8	10
Do not exercise regularly	10	4	14
Totals	**12**	**12**	**24**

Since the number of observations in some of the cells are very small, Chi-square will not yield correct P value, as such Fisher's exact Probability test would be more appropriate and calculated as follows:

$$P = [\{ (12)!\ (12)!\ (10)!\ (14)! \} \ / \ \{ 24 !\ 2!\ 8!\ 10!\ 4! \}]$$

$$= 0.0167$$

Since $P < 0.05$, it indicates that the difference between boys and girls in exercise habits are significantly different.

Analysis of Variance

It is seen that, to test whether the difference in the mean values of two groups of observations could be assumed to be arising out of sampling variation or the two groups are coming out of a common population, t test can be used. When there are more than two groups, to test for the differences in terms of combination of two groups at a time is not appropriate, since the variability present in all the groups is not taken into consideration.

As an example, when antenatal mothers are subjected to different treatments to improve their haemoglobin levels, it can be seen that the total variability in the haemoglobin values of all the antenatal mothers is measured as sum of squares of deviation of the haemoglobin values of all the observations irrespective of the treatment they receive. However, there may be two more types of variability responsible for this total variability, one type of variability may be due to differences in the mothers between the treatment groups, while the second may be due to the differences in the mothers within each of the treatment group. As such three different estimates of the variance of observations can be obtained. First one can be calculated on the basis of all the observations irrespective of the treatment they receive, considering the overall mean, which is the total variability. Another estimate of the variance can be obtained considering the variability between the groups and a third estimate of the variance can be obtained on the basis of the variability within the treatment group. If the variability between mothers treated with different treatments or the variability within each group of treatment are not significantly different, all the above three estimates of variance are unbiased estimates of the population variance, which would be almost same.

With the above considerations, the methodology of Analysis of variance, where the ratio of the variances (F) developed by Fisher, is used to test for the null hypothesis that the mothers of different treatment groups are not significantly varying with their haemoglobin levels and is calculated as :

$$F = \frac{\text{Estimated variance between the groups}}{\text{Estimated variance within the groups}}$$

In other words it can be expressed as

$$F = \frac{\text{Mean sum of squares between groups}}{\text{Mean sum of squares within groups}}$$

If the two variances differ much, the value of 'F' ratio will be high.

The value of 'F' for different degrees of freedom are tabulated as variance ratios. The degrees of freedom are obtained on the basis of the number of groups under comparison and the number of observations in all the groups. The methodology of obtaining such different estimates of variances and testing for their significant difference, applying F test is known as Analysis of Variance (ANOVA).

If the analysis pertains only to testing the difference between groups, then it will be *One Way Analysis of Variance.* If there are more number of factors, within each group, say besides considering only antenatal mothers, if trimester of pregnancy of the antenatal mothers is also considered, analysis can be made to compare the mean difference between treatment groups as well as, between trimester of pregnancy also. Such analysis is known as *Two Way Analysis of Variance.*

The actual computational procedure for an analysis of variance is illustrated in the following example.

a. *One Way Analysis of Variance*

Example 12.7. In a diet survey of antenatal mothers, it was revealed that the iron intake of sample of ten antenatal mothers from each of four villages were as follows. It is desired to find out whether the differences in the mean iron intake between the samples in the four villages are due to chance or can be regarded as statistically significant.

Iron intake in mg			
Village No. 1	Village No. 2	Village No. 3	Village No. 4
11.5	19.5	18.5	30.0
12.5	18.5	16.5	26.5
18.5	16.0	24.5	27.0
21.0	22.0	30.0	34.0
28.0	30.0	28.5	20.0
26.0	24.5	14.0	22.5
14.0	19.0	19.0	28.0
22.0	24.0	17.0	32.0
20.0	19.5	18.0	27.0
22.0	15.0	29.0	25.5
Total 195.5	**208.0**	**215.0**	**272.5**

Various steps in the computations are as follows:

i. Calculate sum of all observation (Σx_{ij}) where x_{ij} represents each observation.

ii. Calculate sum of observations of each village = (T_j)

iii. Calculate sum of squares of all observations = (Σx_{ij}^2)

iv. Calculate total sum of squares:

$= [(\Sigma x_{ij}^{\ 2}) - \{(\Sigma x_{ij})^2 / n \}]$

where n is total number of observations.

The quantity $\{(\Sigma x_{ij})\}^2 / n \}$ is called as correction factor (CF)

v. Calculate ' sum of squares between villages'

$= \{\Sigma (T_j^{\ 2} / k_i) - CF\}$

where T_j is the sum of observations in each village and k_i is the number of observations in each village.

vi. ' Sum of squares within villages' is obtained as difference between the 'Total sum of squares' and the 'Sum of squares between villages'.

Sum of 40 observations

= (11.5 + 12.5 + 18.5 + ...+ 32.0 + 27.0 + 25.5) = 891

Correction factor (CF) = { $(891)^2/40$ } = { 793881/40 }

= 19847.025

'Total sum of squares'

= $(11.5^2 + 12.5^2 + 18.5^2 + ... + 32.0^2 + 27.0^2 + 25.5^2) - CF$

= (21119.5) – (19847.025) = 1272.475

'Sum of squares between villages'

$$= \frac{[(195.5)^2 + (208.0)^2 + (215.0)^2 + (272.5)^2}{10} - 19847.025.$$

as k, no of observations in each village = 10

= (20196.55 – 19847.025) = 349.525

'Sum of squares within villages' =

('Total sum of squares' – 'Sum of squares between villages')

= (1272.475 – 349.525) = 922.950

Degrees of freedom (d.f.) for 'Total sum of squares'.

= (No. of observations – 1) = (40 – 1) =39

Degrees of freedom for ' Sum of squares between villages'

= (No. of villages – 1) = (4 – 1) = 3

Degrees of freedom for 'Sum of squares within villages'.
= (d.f. for Total sum of squares) – (d.f. for Sum of squares between villages)

= (39 – 3) = 36

Mean sum of squares = (Sum of squares/Degrees of freedom)

$$F = \frac{\text{(Mean sum of squares between villages)}}{\text{(Mean sum of squares within villages)}}$$

Analysis of Variance Table

Source of sum of squares	Degree of freedom	Sum of squares	Mean sum of squares	F
Between villages	3	349.525	116.5083	4.544
Within villages	36	922.950	25.6375	
Total	**39**	**1272.475**		

F, which is the variance ratio, is obtained by dividing the 'between villages mean sum of squares' by 'within villages mean sum of squares'.

P value obtained from the variance ratio tables of Fisher and Yates, corresponding to the calculated value of 'F' for the respective degrees of freedom, enables conclusions as to the significance of the differences in the variability between the villages.

From the Variance ratio table, F value corresponding to the (3, 36) degrees of freedom is 4.38, for P = 0.01.

Since the calculated value of F is 4.544 which is more than this tabulated value, it can be concluded that 'between the villages' variation is significant at P < 0.01, meaning thereby that mean iron intake of antenatal mothers in the four villages are significantly different.

The above analysis is the first step in studying the overall differences between the groups. If the analysis of variance suggests significant differences between the groups, it is necessary to examine the group means, the size of differences between the group means and also to see if these differences are significant. Analysis of variance provides an estimate of the standard error to test these differences.

An estimate of the standard error of the differences between the group means is equal to:

$\sqrt{(2s^2/k)}$

Where s^2 is the 'within groups mean sum of squares' and k is the number of observations in each of the group under comparison. If the number of observations are different in the groups, an average of the number of observations in the groups can be taken as an approximate estimate of k.

If the difference between the means of the two groups is more than a quantity $\{t_{0.05} \sqrt{(2s^2/k)}\}$, which is known as the *Least significant difference* (LSD), the group means can be concluded as significantly different at $P < 0.05$.

The quantity $t_{0.05}$ is the value of t statistic corresponding to the degrees of freedom of 'Sum of squares within groups' in the Analysis of variance table, corresponding to $P = 0.05$.

The calculation of Least significance difference is illustrated in the following example.

Example 12.8. Means of the iron intake of antenatal mother of four villages given in Example 12.7 are as follows:

	Villages			
	1	2	3	4
Mean iron intake in mg	19.55	20.80	21.50	27.25

s^2 = 'Within villages mean sum of squares' = 25.6375

k = Number of observations in each village = 10

d.f. of within villages = 36

t statistics value corresponding to P = 0.05 for 36 d.f is 2.03

$$LSD = \{t_{0.05}\sqrt{(2s^2/k)}\}$$

$= (2.03) \times \{\sqrt{(2 \times 25.6375) / 10}\}$

$= (2.03 \times 2.2644)$

$= 4.597$

On the basis of the above value of LSD at P = 0.05, it can be seen that only the mean difference in iron intake of antenatal mothers of village No. 4 is significantly higher than the corresponding differences in the mean iron intake of the mothers in villages 1, 2 and 3, while the other means are not significantly different.

To find the significance of the mean differences between different groups, apart from Least significance difference, there are also other tests like Scheffe's test, Tuckey's test and other sophisticated tests.

In *Scheffe's test* comparisons between the groups are made in terms of F ratio calculated as,

$$F = \frac{(M_1 - M_2)^2}{\{s^2 (n_1 + n_2)\} / (n_1 \, n_2)}$$

Where,

s^2 is the 'Within Mean sum of squares ' obtained in the Analysis of variance and

n_1 and n_2 are the number of observations in the two groups being compared.

Thus in the above Example, comparison between 1st and 2nd village means can be done as follows:

$M_1 = 19.55 \quad M_2 = 20.80$

s^2 = 'Within villages mean sum of squares ' = 25.6375

n_1 and n_2 = Number of observations in each village = 10

$$F = \frac{(19.55 - 20.80)^2}{25.6375\,(10 + 10) / (10 \times 10)}$$

$$= \frac{(1.25)^2}{5.1275}$$

$= 0.3047$

F value for 3 and 36 d.f. is 2.86 at 5% level. This value if multiplied by (k – 1), the degrees of freedom, for 'between villages sum of squares' will be (3 x 2.86) = 8.58. Only if the calculated F ratio, between the two compared villages is above this value, conclusion can be made that the difference between the village means is significantly different at 5% level. Since the calculated value of F between villages 1 and 2 is only 0.3047, it can be concluded that the mean iron consumption by antenatal mothers in the two villages is not significantly different at 5% level.

Similarly significance of differences between means of other villages can also be compared.

b) *Two Way Classification*

In the previous section it was seen that when there are more than two groups, where only a particular characteristic is studied the differences between the groups can be tested using analysis of variance technique. In many experiments, it may be desirable to study the differences within sub classification of groups also. Suppose, in the example illustrated under 12.7, if the iron intake of antenatal mothers in the different villages were studied according to the trimester of the antenatal period also, then one may be interested to look into the significance of differences of mean iron intake both between villages as well as within the trimester of pregnancies. Such analysis can be made by *Analysis of variance using two way classification.*

The computational procedures involved in such an analysis is illustrated through the following example.

Example 12.9. Iron intake of antenatal mothers in different periods of pregnancy in 10 villages.

Ante-period (Trimester)	Villages										Total of each tri-mester (R_i)
	1	2	3	4	5	6	7	8	9	10	
I	11.5	19.5	18.5	12.5	18.5	16.5	26.5	18.5	16.0	24.5	182.5
II	27.0	28.0	22.0	21.0	15.0	19.5	20.0	26.0	30.0	28.5	237.0
III	28.0	30.0	26.0	30.0	24.5	28.5	26.0	30.0	27.0	25.5	275.5
Total of village	**66.5**	**77.5**	**66.5**	**63.5**	**58.0**	**64.5**	**72.5**	**74.5**	**73.0**	**78.5**	**695.0**

Various steps involved in the calculations of 'Total sum of squares' and Correction Factor (CF) and 'Sum of squares between villages' are similar to the one illustrated under Example 12.6.

In this case, the 'Sum of squares between trimesters' is obtained in a similar manner as that of 'Sum of squares between villages'.

Sum of squares between trimesters = $\{\Sigma (R_i^2 / k_i)\} - CF$

$= \{(R_1^2 / k_1) + (R_2^2 / k_2) + (R_3^2 / k_3)\} - CF$

Where, R_i is the sum of all the cases in a row, each trimester, k_i is the number of observations in that particular row (trimester).

Sum of all observations = 695.

Sum of squares (SS) of all observations = 16985.5

Correction factor = $\{(695)^2\} / 30 = 16100.83$

Total sum of squares = (16985.5 – 16100.83) = 884.67

SS between villages

$$= \frac{\{(66.5)^2 + (77.5)^2 \ldots\ldots\ldots\ldots + (78.5)^2\}}{3} - (16100.83)$$

= (48705/3) – (16100.83)

= (16235.0 – 16100.83) = 134.17

SS between Trimesters

$$= \frac{\{(182.5)^2 + (237.0)^2 + (275.5)^2\}}{10} - (16100.83)$$

= (16537.55 – 16100.83) = 436.72

Residual SS = (Total SS) – (SS between villages) – (SS between Trimesters)

Residual df = (df of Total SS) – (df of SS between villages) – (df of SS between Trimesters)

Mean sum of squares = (Sum of squares/Degrees of freedom)

Analysis of Variance Table

Source of SS	df	Sum of squares	MSS	F
Between villages	9	134.17	14.908	0.855
Between Trimesters	2	436.72	218.36	12.526
Residual	18	313.78	17.432	
Total	**29**	**884.67**		

From the table of F values at P = 0.05, it is seen that F value for (9,18) d.f. corresponding to 'Between Villages' is 2.46, while the calculated value is 0. 85 which is less than the Table value.

Table value of F at P = 0.05 for (2,18) d.f. corresponding to 'Between Trimesters' is 3.16, while the corresponding calculated value is 12.526 which is more than the Table value.

From the above values it can be concluded that the differences in the mean iron intake of antenatal mothers between the villages are not significantly different while the differences in the mean iron intake between the trimesters of pregnancy are significantly different. Further analysis to look into the difference within the subgroup means can be done using least significant differences or other tests.

Assumptions Underlying Analysis of Variance

In the application of the above methodologies it is assumed that the effects of the different treatments under comparison are additive and that the error sum of squares are normally and independently distributed with the same variance.

In actual practice the above conditions are rarely fulfilled in complete. However, minor nonconformity to the above assumptions may not affect the results to a great extent. Whenever the above conditions are grossly not fulfilled, certain transformations of the data are available which will make the data more amenable to the analysis and reduce errors of wrong conclusion.

Analysis of Co-variance

In many experiments, the outcome of a variable depends on the magnitude of the variable before subjecting the experimental units for experimentation. As such, it may be necessary to analyse the outcome values in relation to initial values. In some other cases, the outcome of a particular variable may be dependent on the outcome of another variable. In such cases it is desired to analyse the significance of the effect of this variable on the outcome of the experimental variable.

Analysis of co-variance is a technique that enables such analysis. This technique combines features of analysis of variance and regression analysis.

Non Parametric Tests

We have seen that for applying standard error test, t test or Analysis of variance, we assume that the variable is distributed normally and also that there is homogeneity of variances between the groups. But at times we come across variables like rankings, which do not confirm to any probability distribution or may not be distributed normally. In such situation the above tests may not be applicable and we have to use some non-parametric or distribution free tests. Different tests like *The Sign test, Wilcoxon's signed rank test, Mann Whitney test, Kruskal-Wallis H test, Friedman test,* etc. are available for testing of hypothesis in such situations.

a. *The Sign Test*

There are situations where certain codes or ranks are given for the alternatives of a variable and the distribution pattern of these codes may not be explicitly known. As an example, there may be two diagnostic procedures of a disease which are to be tested for their concurrence. The two procedures can be applied on random samples of patients of the disease. The categorisation of the observations can be made in terms of '1' whenever a person is considered as a patient of the particular disease or 'zero' whenever the person is considered as not a patient of the disease, on the basis of diagnostic procedures. Thus there will be two sets of codes in terms of '1' and 'zero' for the two diagnostic procedures. The difference between the two test procedures can be coded in terms of (+) or (–) taking the difference between zero and one, corresponding to the two test procedures applied on a single individual.

The significance of the difference between the two procedures can be tested using the usual χ^2 test, calculated as follows.

$$\chi^2 = \frac{(|\ a - b\ | - 1)^2}{n} \quad \text{with one df}$$

where, 'a' and 'b' are the number of (+) and (–) respectively and n = (a + b)

All zero differences, i.e. when the two tests are identical in their results, are omitted for calculation so that 'n' is always equal to (a + b).

P is obtained from the χ^2 distribution table and the conclusion about the significance is made as usual.

Example 12.10. Twelve patients of clinically diagnosed amoebiasis were administered two diagnostic procedures, one based on serology and the other based on parasitology and results of diagnosis are coded as '1' whenever the case is diagnosed as amoebic and 'zero' whenever not diagnosed. To test whether there is any significant association between the two diagnostic procedures or not. The Sign test is applied as follows.

Patient No.	Serology	Parasitology	Difference
1	1	0	+
2	1	0	+
3	0	1	–
4	1	0	+
5	1	0	+
6	0	0	0
7	1	0	+
8	1	0	+
9	0	0	0
10	0	1	–
11	0	1	–
12	1	1	0

Number of (+) = a = 6

Number of (–) = b = 3

n = (a + b) = 9

The 3 zero differences are omitted

$$\chi^2 = \frac{(|6-3|-1)^2}{9} \text{ with one df}$$

$$= \frac{(3-1)^2}{9} = \frac{4}{9} = 0.444$$

The P value for a $\chi^2 = 0.444$ at one df is more than 0.50. The test indicates that the difference between the two diagnostic procedures is not significant.

b. *Wilcoxon's Signed Rank Test*

This test is useful for testing the significance of differences in paired observations, when the data is quantitative in nature. Here the difference in the paired values of the observations on each unit is ranked according to the size of the difference, irrespective of the fact that the difference is positive or negative. When once they are ranked, then the signs of the original differences are assigned to the ranks. Under the null hypothesis, it is equally likely that any difference can have either (+) or (–). The sum of all the ranks with (+) sign and that of ranks with (–) sign are obtained separately.

The smaller sum out of the above two is referred to the tables prepared by Wilcoxon (Appendix table 6) without considering the sign, against the number of pairs observed. The table gives the maximum rank sum required for rejection of the null hypothesis under different probability levels. So whenever the calculated smaller rank sum value is less than the tabulated rank sum value at 5% level, conclusions are made that the difference between the two groups of observations is significant at 5% level.

While applying the above test, when there are common value for the differences in more than one pair, i.e. there are tied values, then each of the tied difference is assigned the average of the ranks that would be assigned if there is no tie.

When the number of pairs exceeds 16, which is the limit of number of pairs in the tables given by Wilcoxon the normal approximation for getting the probability of rejection of null hypothesis is obtained from the formula:

$Z = (|\mu - T|) - ½) / \sigma$

Where, T = Smaller rank sum

$\mu = n(n+1)/4$

$\sigma = \sqrt{\{((2n+1)\mu / 6\}}$

n = Number of pairs of observations

P is obtained from the Normal distribution table corresponding to the value of calculated Z. As a rule of thumb $Z > 1.96$ signifies rejection of the null hypothesis at $P < 0.05$.

Example 12.11. The serum fibrinogen degradation product (FDP) in microgram/ml in patients who underwent prostate operation were noted before and after operation and are as given below.

Serum FPD values in micro gm/ml				
Case No.	Before operation	After operation	Difference	Signed rank
1	5.0	7.8	– 2.8	– 2
2	10.0	180.0	– 170.0	– 11
3	18.0	10.0	+ 8.0	+ 5
4	5.0	80.0	– 75.0	– 10
5	10.0	15.0	– 5.0	– 3.5
6	20.0	10.0	+ 10.0	+ 6
7	5.0	180.0	– 175.0	–12
8	2.5	40.0	– 37.5	– 8
9	15.0	10.0	+ 5.0	+ 3.5
10	10.0	7.5	+ 2.5	+ 1
11	80.0	10.0	+ 70.0	+ 9
12	5.0	20.0	– 15.0	– 7

To test whether there is any significant difference in the FDP values before and after operation the test is applied as follows.

First the difference between before and after operation values is obtained and these differences are ranked according to their magnitude.

Note that the two values of difference 5, have been given the average of the ranks 3 and 4, i.e. 3.5.

Sum of (+) ranks = 24.5

Sum of (–) ranks = 53.5

From the *Wilcoxon's signed rank test* table it is observed that for 12 pairs, a rank sum of less than or equal to 14 is required for rejection of the null hypothesis at 5% level. Since the calculated rank sum is 24.5 which is more than the tabulated value of 14, the null hypothesis, that the pre and post-operative values of FDP is not significantly different cannot be rejected and as such accepted at $P > 0.05$.

c. *Mann Whitney Test*

This test is useful for testing the differences between unpaired observations. Here the observations are arranged in the order of their magnitude taking observations of both the samples together. Proper tag is made to distinguish the observations of the two samples separately. Then the ranks are assigned to the combined observations according to their magnitude. Whenever there are observations with common magnitude i.e., tied values, average of the ranks is given to them as in the case of Wilcoxon's signed rank test. Then the sum of ranks of each of the samples is calculated separately.

The smaller rank sum out of the above two is referred to the tables prepared by Mann & Whitney (Appendix Table 7) which gives the maximum sum of ranks required for rejection of null hypothesis, under different probability levels. So whenever the calculated smaller rank sum is less than the tabulated value, the null hypothesis is rejected. When the two samples are of unequal size the smaller rank sum is computed as:

$$T_2 = n_1 (n_1 + n_2 + 1) - T_1$$

Where T_1 is the rank sum of the sample with smaller number of observations, while n_1 and n_2 are the number of observations in the two samples, T, the smaller of T_1 and T_2 is referred to in the above mentioned table. Usually when the values of n_1 and n_2 are greater than 20, Normal approximation is followed and Z is calculated using the formula:

$$Z = (|\mu - T|) - ½) / \sigma$$

$$\mu = n_1 (n_1 + n_2 + 1) / 2$$

$$\sigma = \sqrt{(n_2 \mu / 6)}$$

where n_1 is the smaller sample size and n_2 is the bigger sample size. The calculated value is referred to the tables of Normal distribution and P value is obtained.

Example 12.12. A sample of patients who underwent prostate operation were treated with a drug to reduce the serum fibrinogen degradation production (FDP) while another sample of such patients were kept as a control group without any drug.

To test whether there is any significant difference between the two groups in the FDP values, Mann–Whitney test is applied as follows:

FDP values in micro gm/ml								
Control group	10.0	180.0	80.0	5.0	40.0	15.0	30.0	160.0
Treated group	7.8 5.0	40.0 7.5	10.0	80.0	180.0	5.0	80.0	10.0

FDP values of both the groups are arranged in the order of magnitude with their ranks.

FDP Value	**5.0**	5.0	5.0	7.5	7.8	**10.0**	10.0	10.0	**15.0**	**30.0**
Ranks	**2**	2	2	4	5	**7**	7	7	**9**	**10**
FDP Values	**40.0**	40.0	**80.0**	80.0	80.0	**160.0**	**180.0**	180.0		
Ranks	**11.5**	11.5	**14**	14	14	**16**	**17.5**	17.5		

To facilitate tagging the sample values with their ranks of control group are given in bold font.

Note that the ranks are tied with reference to the following common observations.

5.0   10.0   40.0   80.0   180.0

Since the size of the two samples are different, first the sum of ranks T_1 of the smaller sample is found out.

$T_1 = 2 + 7 + 9 + 10 + 11.5 + 14 + 16 + 17.5 = 87$

$T_2 = n_1(n_1 + n_2 + 1) - T_1$

where n_1 is the smaller sample size and n_2 the bigger sample size

$T_2 = 8\ (8 + 10 + 1) - 87 = (8 \times 19) - 87 = 65$

Since 65 is smaller than 87 we refer to this value in the table to obtain P value.

$T = 65$, $n_1 = 8$ and $n_2 = 10$

The table value of T corresponding to these degrees of freedom is 53, at P = 0.05 which is less than the calculated value of 65. This suggests that the null hypothesis cannot be rejected. The obvious conclusion would be that the treated and the control groups are not significantly different with respect to FDP values.

d. *Kruskal-Wallis H test*

In contrast to F test which is a parametric test, used in Analysis of variance, Kruskal-Wallis H test is a non parametric analysis of variance in one way classification. This test is used to test whether or not the groups of independent samples have been drawn from the same population.

This test is calculated from the formula,

$$H = \frac{12}{n\ (n+1)} \{\Sigma(R_i^{\ 2} / n_i)\} - 3\ (n+1)$$

where, n is the Total No. of observations in all the samples together,

R_i is the sum of ranks in the ith sample,

n_i is the number of observations in the ith sample.

H test is interpreted as chi-square with degrees of freedom equal to one less than the number of groups compared.

Calculation of the test is illustrated in the following example.

Example 12.13. Scores obtained by three groups of caretakers of chronically ill patients, on the burden of disease felt by them, are given below. To test whether there is any significant difference in the scores of the three groups, the test is applied as follows.

Group 1		Group 2		Group 3	
Score	Rank	Score	Rank	Score	Rank
10	1	11	2	30	20
12	3	14	4	32	22
15	5	22	12	24	14
17	7	28	18	31	21
23	13	20	10	26	16
18	8	16	6	34	24
19	9	29	19	27	17
		21	11	33	23
				25	15
$n_1 = 7$	$R_1 = 46$	$n_2 = 8$	$R_2 = 82$	$n_3 = 9$	$R_3 = 172$

All the observations are ranked in ascending order of their magnitude irrespective of their groups. Tied observations are ranked as already explained in the previous test. Then the sum of ranks in each group is calculated.

n = total no. of observations = 24

$$- \{12 / (24 \times 25)\} \{ (\frac{(46)^2}{7} + \frac{(82)^2}{8} + \frac{(172)^2}{9} \} - 3\ (24 + 1)$$

$$= (0.02)\ (302.29 + 840.50 + 3287.11) - 75$$

$$= 13.60$$

Here the degrees of freedom = 2

For d.f.= 2, chi square value at P = 0.01, is 9.210 and since the calculated value is 13.60, P value is less than 0.05 which indicates that the differences are not due to sampling variation and hence is significant at 5% level or in other words the samples are not from the same population.

e. *Friedman Test*

In the above example given under Kruskal-Wallis H test, there was only one variable group which was being compared. There may be investigations, where each group may have further subdivisions as in the case of Two-way Analysis of variance. In situations where doubts exist about the parametric assumptions of normality and homogeneity of variances, Friedman test can be applied to test whether the samples have been drawn from the same population or not.

For applying this test the responses of each observation is arranged into rows and columns, where rows represent the groups and columns represent the subdivisions in each group. Observations in each group, i.e. each row are ranked in either increasing or decreasing order, starting from 1. Then the sum of ranks corresponding to each column is calculated.

The test statistic is calculated with the null hypothesis that the rank totals in each column do not differ significantly.

The test statistic is calculated from the formula:

$\chi^2 = [\{(12)\ (\Sigma\ R_j)^2\ \}\ /\ \{nk\ (k + 1)\ \}] - \{3\ n\ (k + 1)\}$

where ΣR_j is the sum of ranks in each column

n is the number of rows

k is the number of columns.

Normally, the test statistic follows a χ^2 distribution with (k – 1) degrees of freedom, when the number of rows and columns are less, special tables devised by *Siegal* can also be used to find the probability level of rejection of null hypothesis. In the following example application of this test is illustrated.

Example 12.14. The data pertains to scores obtained by three groups of caregivers on the rehabilitation needs perceived by them according to the domain of need.

To test whether the three groups are significantly same with regards to these scores for different domains the test is applied as follows.

Group of care givers	Need 1		Need 2		Need 3		Need 4	
	Score	Rank	Score	Rank	Score	Rank	Score	Rank
Group I	13	**2**	9	**4**	10	**3**	16	**1**
Group II	10	**2**	4	**3**	3	**4**	12	**1**
Group III	12	**1**	6	**3**	2	**4**	10	**2**
Rank sums		**5**		**10**		**11**		**4**

The scores obtained for the needs in each group are ranked in order within each group.

Ranks within each column are totalled up to get ΣR_j for each column.

n = No. of groups = 3

k = No. of columns = 4

$(\Sigma R_j)^2 = (5^2 + 10^2 + 11^2 + 4^2) = 262$

Substituting these values in the formula,

$\chi^2 = [(12)(262)] / \{(3 \times 4)(4 + 1)\}] - \{(3)(3)(4 + 1)\}$

$= [(3144) / (60)] - (45)$

$= (52.4) - (45) = 7.4$

Degrees of freedom = k – 1 = 4 – 1 = 3

From table, for 3 d.f., and $\chi^2 = 7.4$ P value is between 0.10 and 0.05, as such null hypothesis is accepted and concluded that there is no significant difference in the needs felt by the three groups.

13
Chapter

Correlation and Regression

Meaning and Definition of Correlation

When dealing with two sets of variables measured on the same unit, it may so happen that one variable may be in a way related to the other. That is to say that with the change in one variable from one value to the other, the other variable will also change in its value corresponding to the change in the first variable. Then it is assumed that there is a correlation between the two variables. This correlation may be either due to some direct relationship between the two variables or due to some inherent factor common to both the variables. The quantum of this correlation is measured in terms of *Correlation Coefficient*. This measure takes into consideration the co-variation between the two variables in relation to the variation within the two variables.

As an example, considering the correlation of height and weight of children up to 15 years, it may be observed that the weight increases with the increase in the height. It is possible to measure the degree of relationship between the height and weight of these children in terms of a correlation coefficient.

Scatter Diagram

Before calculating the correlation coefficient an approximate idea about the extent and type of relationship between the two variables can be known by plotting the variables into a scatter diagram as described in Chapter 6. In this diagram one variable is represented on the X-axis while the other on the Y-axis and each pair of observation is plotted as a dot. The diagram will be a scatter of dots. Three different types of scatter diagrams are given in Figure 13.1.

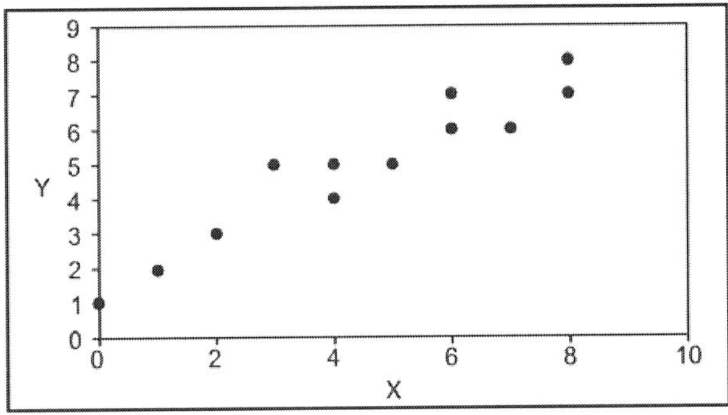

Fig. 13.1: Scatter diagram showing positive correlation

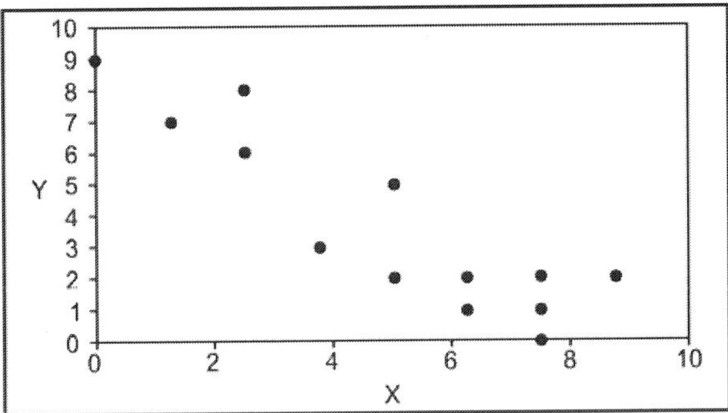

Fig. 13.2: Scatter diagram showing negative correlation

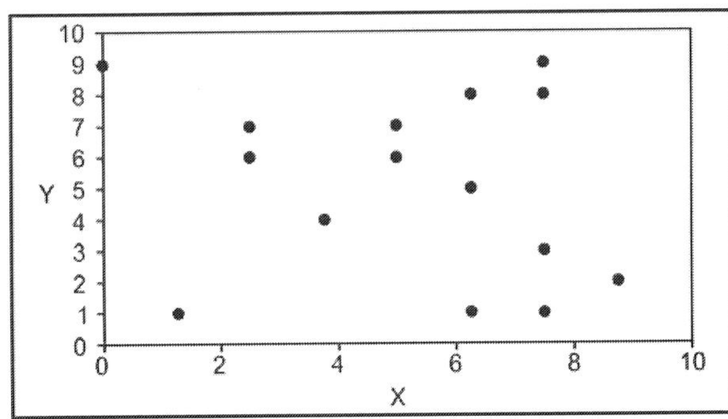

Fig. 13.3: Scatter diagram showing no correlation

In the first scatter diagram, Figure 13.1, it can be seen that the high values of X are associated with high values of Y and low values of X with low values of Y.

In the second scatter diagram, Figure 13.2, high values of X are associated with low values of Y and low values of Y with high values of X.

In the third scatter diagram, Figure 13.3, it seems that there is no association between the values of X and Y and the points are highly scattered.

First and second scatter diagrams suggest that there is some correlation between the variables X and Y while the third scatter diagram suggests that there is no correlation between X and Y.

The correlation shown in the first scatter diagram is a positive correlation, i.e. with the increase in the value of X, value of Y is also increasing and that of second scatter diagram is a negative correlation, i.e. with the increase in X value, value of Y is decreasing.

Covariance

The amount of covariation between any two variables is measured in terms of *covariance* calculated by the formula.

$$\text{Cov}\ (x_1x_2) = [\Sigma(x_1\ x_2) - (\Sigma x_1\ \Sigma x_2)/n]/(n-1)$$

Where $\Sigma(x_1\ x_2)$ is the sum of the products of the values of the variables in each pair, $\Sigma\ x_1$ and $\Sigma\ x_2$, are the sum of values of each of the variables, while n is the number of pairs of observations.

Correlation Coefficient

The degree of correlation between two variables is measured in terms of correlation coefficient represented by 'r', when at least one of the variables is distributed normally. This correlation coefficient is called as the product-moment correlation coefficient. For calculation of this quantity, the co-variation between the two variables is considered in relation to the variation of each of the variables within itself. It is seen that the covariance gives the covariation between the variables, while the variance or standard deviation gives the variation of a variable within itself.

The formula for the calculation of correlation coefficient is given by

$$r = \frac{\text{Covariance between two variables}}{(\text{SD of first variable}) \times (\text{SD of second variable})}$$

Mathematically, if x_1, and x_2, are two variables with n pairs of observations then,

$$r = \frac{[\Sigma(x_1\ x_2)\ n\ (\Sigma x_1\ \Sigma x_2)\ /\ n]}{\sqrt{[\{(\Sigma x_1^{\ 2} - (\Sigma x_1)^2\ /\ n)\}\ \{(\Sigma x_2^{\ 2} - (\Sigma x_2)^2 /\ n)\}]}}$$

Range and Interpretation of Correlation Coefficient

i. The correlation coefficient can be either positive or negative depending upon the covariance between the two variables as seen in Figures 13.1 and 13.2.
ii. The correlation coefficient is zero when there is no co-variation between the two variables as seen in scatter diagram of Figure 13.3.
iii. When the relationship is perfect, the correlation coefficient will be either +1 or –1.
iv. Therefore the range of correlation coefficient is from – 1 to +1.
v. The correlation coefficient is also subject to sampling variation and hence observed value of 'r' is to be tested for its significance.
vi. The standard error of correlation coefficient is given by $\sqrt{\ [(1-r^2)\ /\ (n-2)]}$ where r is the correlation coefficient and n is the number of pairs of observations.
vii. The test of significance for correlation coefficient is given by

$$t = r\ /\ \sqrt{\ [\ (1-r^2)\ /\ (n-2)]} \quad \text{with } (n-2) \text{ df}$$

The corresponding probability level of significance is worked out from t-distribution table.

Calculation of Correlation Coefficient for Ungrouped Data

For an ungrouped data, the correlation coefficient is calculated directly from the formula given earlier. Various steps involved in the calculation are as follows :

i. First, find the product of x_1, and x_2 for each set of observations and get the sum of these products, $\Sigma(x_1 x_2)$.

ii. Compute the sum of first variable as well as the second variable separately and get (Σx_1) and (Σx_2)

iii. The numerator is obtained by substituting these values in formula .

$[\Sigma(x_1 x_2) - (\Sigma x_1 \Sigma x_2) / n]$

iv. Find the square of each of the observation in both the sets and get their sum Σx_1^2 and Σx_2^2.

v. Square the sums obtained in step (ii) for each of x_1 and x_2 and divide by n to get $(\Sigma x_1)^2 / n$ and $(\Sigma x_2)^2 / n$

vi. Denominator is obtained by substituting the values obtained in step (iv) and (v) in the formula

$$\sqrt{[(\Sigma x_1^2 - (\Sigma x_1)^2 / n)][(\Sigma x_2^2 - (\Sigma x_2)^2 / n)]}$$

vii. r is obtained by dividing the result of step (iii) by step (vi).

Example 13.1. Following data gives the age of the mother in years at the time of delivery and weight of the newborn in sample of deliveries.

Age of the Mother (x_1)	25	36	25	28	30	22	35	30	21	20	41	35	30	20	20
Weight of the new-born in lbs (x_2)	5.0	8.0	7.0	7.5	7.5	6.0	7.0	7.0	5.2	6.1	8.0	7.0	7.0	4.5	4.0

In order to quantify the relationship between the two variables, age of the mother (x_1) and the weight of the newborn (x_2), correlation coefficient can be obtained by calculating the following quantities from the data.

$\Sigma x_1 = 418$	$(\Sigma x_1)^2 = 174724$
$\Sigma x_2 = 96.8$	$(\Sigma x_2)^2 = 9370.24$
$\Sigma x_1^2 = 12286.00$	$\Sigma x_2^2 = 647.00$

$\Sigma (x_1 x_2) = 2794.2$ $\quad\quad$ $n=15$

$(\Sigma x_1)^2 / n = 11648.27$

$(\Sigma x_2)^2 / n = 624.68$

$[(\Sigma x_1) (\Sigma x_2) / n)] = (418) \times (96.8) / 15$

$= 40462.4/15 = 2697.5$

$[\Sigma (x_1 x_2) - (\Sigma x_1) (\Sigma x_2) / n] = (2794.2) - (2697.5)$

$= 96.7$

$[\Sigma x_1^2 - (\Sigma x_1)^2 / n] = (12286.00 - 11648.27) = 637.73$

$[\Sigma x_2^2 - (\Sigma x_2)^2 / n] = (647.00 - 624.68) = 22.32$

$\sqrt{} \; [\{(\Sigma x_1^2 - (\Sigma x_1)^2 / n) \}\{(\Sigma x_2^2 - (\Sigma x_2)^2 / n) \}]$

$= \sqrt{} [(637.73) (22.32)] = \sqrt{} (14234.1336) = 119.31$

$$r = \frac{[\Sigma x_1 \; x_2 \; n \, (\Sigma x_1 \; \Sigma x_2 \, / \, n)]}{\sqrt{\;} \; [\{(\Sigma x_1^2 \; n \, (\Sigma x_1)^2 \, / \, n)\} \, \{(\Sigma x_2^2 \; n(\Sigma x_2)^2 \, / \, n)\}]}$$

$= (96.7) / (119.31) = 0.81$

For testing the significance of this calculated r, first standard error of r is calculated from the formula and then t test is applied.

$= \sqrt{} [(1 - r^2) / (n - 2)] = \sqrt{} [(1 - 0.6561) / 13]$

$= \sqrt{} [(0.3439) / 13] = \sqrt{} (0.0265) = 0.163$

$t = r / \sqrt{} [(1 - r^2) / (n - 2)] = (0.81) / (0.163) = 4.97$

From t-distribution table, the value of P for t = 4.97 at 13 d.f. is less than 0.01 which shows that there is a positive significant correlation between the age of the mother and the weight of the newborn.

Linear Regression

In the case of correlation, it was seen that the degree of correlation between the two variables could be measured using the correlation coefficient. In some cases if this correlation is due to a latent factor associated with both the variables, then the correlation is known as *'Spurious correlation'*. In some other cases, it may be that one of the variables directly causes the change in the other variable as already explained. In the latter case, the variable, which causes the change, is known as the independent variable. The height and weight of children given in the case of correlation is an example for this. In this case a change in the independent variable height of the child will cause a change in the dependant variable weight of the child.

The change of dependent variable with respect to change in the independent variable is known as Regression.

Regression coefficient is an estimate of the amount of change in the dependant variable for a unit change in the independent variable. This quantity is represented by 'b'.

Linear Regression Equation

The relationship between the two variables can be represented by a mathematical equation known as *Regression Equation.* A regression line can be plotted when the relationship is linear i.e., the dependant variable either increases or decreases throughout with the change in the independent variable in a linear manner, the equation will be of the type, $y = (a + b\,x)$

Where, y is the dependent variable
x is the independent variable
b is the regression coefficient
a represents the value of y for x = 0, which is also known as y intercept.

In the above linear equation the regression coefficient b is calculated from the formula.

$$b = \frac{\Sigma xy - [(\Sigma x)(\Sigma y) / n]}{[\Sigma x^2 - (\Sigma x)^2 / n]}$$

Where, b is the regression coefficient of independent variable x, upon dependant variable y .

After testing for the significance of regression coefficient, the linear regression line of y upon x can be fitted in the form

$$y = (a + bx)$$

by substituting the various values calculated, in the formula

$$y = \bar{y} + (x - \bar{x})\,b$$

Where, $\bar{y}$ and $\bar{x}$ are the means of the variable y and x and b is the calculated regression coefficient.

The above regression equation can be used for estimating values of dependant variable y for various values of independent variable within the range covered by the two variables in the given sample of observations.

Interpretation of Linear Regression

i Linear regression equation should be used for estimating the values of dependant variable, only when a straight line fully answers the relationship.

ii The regression line should not be extended beyond the values of the variable for which they are plotted.

iii Whenever there is correlation, it does not mean that there is also a regression. The correlation may be due to inherent factor acting on both variables and so there may not be any regression at all.

iv The regression coefficient should be tested for significance.

v The standard error of regression coefficient is given by

$$S_b = (S_{y.x}) / \sqrt{\ }\{(\Sigma x^2 - (\Sigma x)^2 / n\}$$

where

$$S_{y.x} = \sqrt{\ }[(1/(n-2)\{\Sigma y^2 - (\Sigma y)^2 / n) - \frac{(\Sigma xy - (\Sigma x)(\Sigma y)/n)^2}{\Sigma x^2 - (\Sigma x)^2 / n}\}]$$

(vi) The regression coefficient is to be tested for null hypothesis using t distribution where

$t = (b / S_b)$ with $(n - 2)$ d.f.

(vii) The standard error of the estimated value of y from the regression equation is given by the quantity $(S_{y.x} / \sqrt{n})$ where $S_{y.x}$ is obtained as above.

Example 13.2. Regression co-efficient and the regression line for the data given in example 13.1 is worked out below using the notation x and y for the age of the mother and weight of the new born respectively in place of x_1 and x_2.

$\Sigma x = 418$ $\bar{x} = 27.9$

$[\Sigma x^2 - (\Sigma x)^2/n] = 637.73$

$\Sigma y = 96.8$ $\bar{y} = 6.45$

$[\Sigma y^2 - (\Sigma y)^2/n] = 22.23$

$[\Sigma xy - (\Sigma x)(\Sigma y)/n] = 96.7$

Regression coefficient of x on y

$$b = \frac{\Sigma xy - [(\Sigma x)(\Sigma y)/n]}{[(\Sigma x^2 - (\Sigma x)^2/n)]}$$

$= (96.7) / (637.73) = 0.152$

The significance of this regression coefficient is worked out by the formula given under (vi) in page number 165 i.e.

$$S_{y.x}{}^2 = \{1/(n-2)\,[\Sigma y^2 - (\Sigma y)^2/n)] - \frac{[\Sigma xy - (\Sigma x)(\Sigma y)/n]^2}{[\Sigma x^2 - (\Sigma x)^2/n)]}\}$$

$S_{y.x} = \sqrt{[\,(1/13)\,\{\,(22.32) - (96.7)^2/(637.73)\}]} = 0.77$

$S_b = (0.77/637.73) = (0.001203)$

$t = 0.152/0.0012 = 126.7$

P value corresponding to a t-value of 126.7 at 13 df is less than 0.001, which shows that the regression coefficient is significant.

The linear regression line is obtained as

$y = \bar{y} + b(x - \bar{x})$

$= 6.45 + 0.152\,(x - 0\ 27.9)$

$= 6.45 + 0.152\,x - 4.24$

$= 2.21 + 0.152\,x.$

Non-linear Regression

In the previous sections, it was seen that if the dependant variable either increases or decreases in equal quantities, throughout the range, with the independent variable, then the regression is linear and can be represented by a linear relationship. Unlike this, it may happen that the dependant variable increases for each change of the independent variable up to a certain value and then it may start decreasing with the change in the independent variable. The reverse process may also happen. In such cases the regression is said to be non-linear. This type of relationship is often seen with the prevalence of certain diseases in different age groups. For example, it is observed that the tuberculosis infection rate in community rises with the age up to a certain age and then starts decreasing with the increase in the age after reaching a maximum at certain age group. This may be due to immunity attained by the community by the time they reach a certain age.

In such a case the relationship is said to be quadratic. The relationship may be of other higher degrees also. In all these cases the equation of the relationship between the two variables are obtained by suitable mathematical procedures.

Multiple Correlation and Regression

In bivariate correlation, it was seen that there will be one dependent variable and only one independent variable which may be related with the dependant variable. But it may happen that there may be more than one independent variable for the causation of the dependant variable. As an example if the weight of a baby at birth is considered, the birth weight may be related to many factors such as age of the mother, period of gestation of the mother at the time of birth, parity of delivery, health condition of the mother and so on. If the overall correlation of all these independent factors with the dependant factor is considered then it is known as *Multiple correlation.*

The multiple correlation coefficient is represented by R and can be estimated by simple correlation coefficients between various variables.

R has no sign since the correlation may be positive with one variable and may be negative with the other. R approaches unity as more and more variables responsible for the causation of the dependent variable are considered.

If an equation is fitted to estimate the dependant variable say the weight of a baby at birth in terms of the other independent variables such as the above factors then the equation is called as the multiple regression equation. If all the pertinent variables are included in the fitting of Multiple regression equation then perfect estimates of the dependant variable can be made from the fitted Regression equation. R approaches unity as more and more variables responsible for the causation of the dependent variable are considered.

The multiple regression equation for the birth weight of a baby in terms of say three quantitative factors like age of the mother, parity of delivery and total calorie intake of food during third trimester of pregnancy will be in the form of,

$$y = a + b_1 x_1 + b_2 x_2 + b_3 x_3$$

Where,

y is the value of weight of the baby at birth

x_1 is the age of the mother

x_2 is the parity of delivery,

x_3 is the total calorie intake of food during third trimester of pregnancy

b_1 is the regression coefficient of y with x_1, when the effect of x_2 and x_3 are held constant, similarly b_2 and b_3 are regression coefficients of y with x_2 and x_3 respectively when the other two variables are held constant and 'a' is a hypothetical value of y when x_1, x_2 and x_3 are zero.

Partial Correlation

It was seen that the dependant variable can be expressed as an equation in terms of the independent variable. When only one independent variable say x_1 is considered and a simple regression equation for y in terms of x_1 is fitted, then the estimates of y for various values of x_1 can be obtained. There may be another variable x_2 on which y is dependent. If a regression equation of y in terms of x_1 and x_2 is fitted, then the precision of the estimates of y obtained in terms of x_1, and x_2 will be better than the precision of estimate y, obtained in terms of x_1 only. If there are more independent variables causing the dependent variable, by inclusion of these variables in the regression equation, precision of the estimate of y can be further improved.

In other words, the difference in variations between the actual values of y and the corresponding estimated values can be made smaller and smaller by the consideration of additional variables which may be responsible for the causation of y.

An estimate of reduction in the variation between the actual and estimated values of y obtained by addition of another variable is measured in terms *Partial correlation coefficient* attributable to this new variable. In other words, the partial correlation coefficient gives a ratio of additional variation answered in estimates of dependent variable, by inclusion of another independent variable, to the unanswered variation before the inclusion of this variable.

Thus the purpose of calculation of the partial correlation coefficient is to analyse the relative importance of the different independent variables in estimating the dependant variable.

As in the case of simple correlation coefficient, the significance of the partial correlation coefficient should also be tested before making conclusions.

The symbolic presentation of partial correlation coefficient is $r_{12..3}......_{n}$, which means the partial correlation coefficient of variables 1 and 2 holding the effect of variables 3 to n constant. This is (n–2)th order partial correlation coefficient. Thus $r_{12..3}$ is the first order partial correlation coefficient between three variables which gives the partial correlation coefficient of variables 1 and 2 holding the effect of variable 3 constant. Similarly when there are four variables, $r_{12.34}$ is the second order partial correlation coefficient between the variables 1 and 2 holding the effects of variables 3 and 4 constant.

Any of the first order partial correlation coefficient can calculated by the formula,

$$r_{12..3} = (r_{12} - r_{13}\, r_{23}) \;/\; \sqrt{\{ (1 - r^2_{13})\, (1 - r^2_{23}) \}}$$

Where r_{12} is the simple correlation coefficient between variable 1 and 2. Similarly r_{13} and r_{23} are respectively the correlation coefficient between the variables 1 and 3, 2 and 3.

Similarly the second order partial correlation coefficient is calculated from the formula,

$$r_{12.34} = (r_{12.4} - r_{13.4}\, r_{23.4}) / \sqrt{\{(1 - r^2_{13.4})(1 - r^2_{23.4})\}}$$

Where the first order partial correlation coefficients are utilised for the calculation.

To test for the significance of partial correlation coefficient the procedure is similar to that of simple correlation coefficient but the degrees of freedom will be (n – 3) for first order coefficient and (n – 4) for second order coefficients and so on.

Similarly the other second order partial correlation coefficients like $r_{13.23}$ or $r_{12.24}$ etc. can be calculated by the substitution of the appropriate partial correlation coefficient in the formula.

Thus a general formula for the calculation of partial correlation coefficient of any order is given by

$$r_{1n.23\ldots(n-1)} = \frac{[(r_{1n.23\ldots\ldots(n-2)}] - [\{r_{1(n-1).23\ldots\ldots(n-2)}\}\{r_{n\,(n-1).23\ldots\ldots(n-2)}\}]}{\sqrt{[1 - r^2_{(n-1).23\ldots(n-2)}][1 - r^2_{[n\,(n-1).23\ldots\ldots(n-2)}]}}$$

Spearman's Rank Correlation Coefficient

It was seen that for the calculation of product-moment correlation coefficient, at least one of the variables is to be distributed normally. In cases where it is not so or when the measurements are in terms of certain ranks and not in exact quantitative terms, then *Spearman's rank correlation coefficient* is calculated. In situations, where original series is in quantitative data but not normally distributed then also this measure of correlation is useful. In this case, one of the series is arranged in the order of magnitude and ranked from 1 to n while the values of the other variable is arranged correspondingly and ranks are assigned and the correlation coefficient of these two rankings is calculated in the usual way. But a simplified formula can be used as,

$$r_{rank} = 1 - [6 \Sigma D^2 / n (n^2 - 1)]$$

Where D is the difference in the ranks of each pair of data and n is the number of pairs of observations.

Whenever there is a tie in the ranks then for each of the tied pairs average of the ranks is assigned.

The range for rank correlation coefficient is also between –1 and +1.

Example 13.4. The performance of seven outpatient departments in a hospital as ranked by two independent judges is as given below.

Out-patient Dept.	Ranking		Difference in ranks	
	Judge I	Judge II	D	D^2
1. Surgery	1	3	-2	4
2. Medicine	2	2	0	0
3. Paediatrics	3	4	-1	1
4. Orthopaedics	4	1	3	9
5. Eye	5	7	-2	4
6. Gynaecology	6	6	0	0
7. ENT	7	5	+2	4

The calculation of rank correlation coefficient between the opinions of the two judges is calculated as follows—

$\Sigma D^2 = 22, \quad n = 7$

$r_{rank} = 1 - [(6 \times 22)/[7 \times (49 - 1)]$

$= (1 - 0.39) = + 0.61$

i.e., correlation coefficient between the rankings of the out patient departments by the two judges is + 0.61.

From the table for testing the significance of rank correlation coefficient given below, it is evident that this value of rank correlation coefficient is not significant as a minimum value of 0.750 is required for significance at 5% level for 7 pairs.

This means that the two judges are not similar in the ranking of the outpatient departments.

For samples of size over 10 pairs the significance level of r_{rank} can be calculated similar to that of r, but for samples of size 10 or less number of pairs, it is given by the following table given by Kendall.

Size of the sample	5% level	1% level
4 or less	None	None
5	1.000	None
6	0.886	1.000
7	0.750	0.893
8	0.714	0.857
9	0.683	0.883
10	0.648	0.794
11	Use tables of significance of r	

Logistic Regression

When dependent variable (outcome variable) happens to be binary in nature viz. an event occurring or not, taking the values unity or zero, the assumption necessary for fitting multiple linear regression model of the type Y = $\alpha + \sum_{i=1}^{k} \beta_i X_i$, is violated as it is unreasonable to assume that distribution of errors as normal. For such data, instead of multiple linear regression analysis, *multiple linear logistic regression (LR)* analysis is used as a multivariate procedure. The main difference between LR and multiple linear regression models is that instead of using the dependent variable as such, we develop a model based on the logit transformation of the dependent variable to satisfy the needed assumptions. Thus, in LR model we predict the probability (p) of an individual with that characteristic for any combination of the explanatory variables. The logistic regression involves modeling the log odds of disease of risk factors comprising the main exposure (s) of interest and potential confounders. The model takes the general form:

$$\text{logit p (Y = 1/X) = logit p} = \log_e (p/1-p) = \alpha + \sum_{i=1}^{k} \beta_i X_i$$

The above model enables us to estimate the probability of happening of an event (Y = 1/X):

$$p\ (Y = 1/X) = \exp\left(\alpha + \sum_{i=1}^{k} \beta_i X_i\right) / [1 + \exp\left(\alpha + \sum_{i=1}^{k} \beta_i X_i\right)]$$

Where p (Y = 1/X) denotes the disease probability in stratum i for an individual with set of regression variables X_i, α is a constant term and represents the log odds of the disease risk for a person with standard set when all the regression variables are zero (X=0). The β's are regression coefficients and indicates the fraction by which the risk is increased (or decreased) for every unit change in X_i and exponential of β_i represents the odds ratio (OR).

The model relates a dichotomous outcome variable (which is assigned a value of 1 if individual develops a disease) to a series of 'k' known regression variables as well as possible confounding and effect modification (interaction) variables. The collection of k regression variables or risk factors is called as covariates or explanatory variables. The model can be modified to allow for multiple (k) levels of main exposure by including (k-1) indicator variables.

Estimation of the Parameters

The unknown parameters in the model α and β_i are estimated using the method of maximum likelihood estimation (MLE). Initially a likelihood function is developed for expressing the probability of observed data with the covariates as a function of unknown parameters. The coefficients in the likelihood function are selected to maximize the value of the function. It maximizes the probability of obtaining the observed data and iterative algorithm is necessary for parameter estimation as the logistic regression model is non-linear.

Fitting of Model

The likelihood inference typically proceeds by fitting a "nested hierarchy of models" each one containing the last. Initially one might start with the model;

$$\text{Logit } p\ (Y = 1/X) = \alpha \text{ or prob of event} = \exp \alpha/(1+ \exp \alpha) \quad ...(1)$$

Which specifies that the disease probabilities do not depend on the regression variables, i.e. the log odds ratio for different X's is zero.

This model will be elaborated in a second model;

Logit p (Y = 1/X) = $\alpha + \beta_1 - X_1$ ...(2)

For which the log odds ratio associated with risk factor X_1 is allowed to be non-zero. A further generalisation for two variables is;

Logit p (Y = 1/X) = $\alpha_1 + \beta_1 X_1 + \beta_2 X_2$ ...(3)

In which the coefficients for two more variables are allowed to be non-zero. At each stage we obtain MLE's of the coefficients in the model, together with their estimated variance and covariance's. Thus, the model can be generalized for "k" variables.

Logit p (Y = 1/X) = $\alpha_1 + \beta_1 X_1 + \beta_2 X_2 + ... + \beta_k X_k$ or

Probability of an event = exp Z/(1 + exp Z)

where Z = $\alpha_1 + \beta_1 X_1 + \beta_2 X_2 + ... + \beta_k X_k$

Goodness of Fit of the Model

Likelihood ratio test: One of the methods of assessing the goodness of fit of the model is actually to examine how likely the sample results are predicted when the parameter estimates are substituted. This is done using a likelihood ratio test. It is simply the difference of the maximized log likelihood statistics for the two models without and with the variables, which is distributed as a Chi-square statistic.

The probability of observed results given the parameter estimate is known as likelihood. Since the likelihood is a small number less than 1, it is customary to use -2 times the log of the likelihood (-2LL) as a measure to test the model, which has a Chi-square distribution with "r" degrees of freedom. If a model fits perfectly, the log likelihood is 'one' and -2 times the log likelihood is zero.

Hypothesis Testing About Coefficients

Test based on Wald statistics

Test for the significance of the parameters in a model is simply to compare their estimated values against zero, using their standard errors as a reference. For large sample sizes the test that a coefficient is zero is based on Wald statistics, which has a Chi-square distribution. When a variable has a single degree of freedom, the Wald statistics is just the square of the ratio of the coefficient to its standard error. The differences in the likelihood statistics with and without the variable are also used as a test for the significance of additional parameters in the model.

14 Chapter Demography

Definition and Uses

The word Demography has been coined from the Greek words 'Demos' and "Graphy' which means 'Population' and 'Science'. As such demography is a science of studying population and related aspects. The three components of demographic change are births, deaths and migration. In other words, during a period of time population may change due to four factors, birth of a person may take place in the area, a resident in the area may die, an outsider may move into the area and a resident may move out of the area. Demography deals with a study of the above factors along with the associated social factors like marriage, occupation, literacy and so on.

Demographic studies in terms of various population characteristics are useful to ascertain :

i. Quantum and distribution of people residing within an area.
ii. To describe past growth, decline and dispersal of population as accurately as possible.
iii. To understand the casual relations between the population trends and different aspects of social organisation.
iv. To make predictions of future developments and their possible implications.

With the present day population explosion in our country it is important to study these aspects for better planning of our health and other developmental activities.

Stages of Demographic Evolution

From the study of the population changes in the past and in the light of the variables affecting the population change, five possibilities for the stages of population change can be considered.

i. When both birth and death rates are high and are almost equal the net resultant change in the population neutralises and the total population tends to be almost stationary, this stage is termed as *high stationary stage.*

ii. With the advancements in medical and health facilities, the death rate begins to fall. However with the prevailing customs and mores not permitting adoption of birth control measures, the birth rate will be either increasing or stationary thus resulting in a population explosion. This stage is known as *early expanding stage.*

iii. With further developments in medical and health technology and awareness amongst the population about ill effects of population explosion, the death rate falls steeply and the birth rate tends to come down slowly when the population increase may slow down but still the growth rate remaining at a higher level. This stage is known as *late expanding stage.*

iv. With the awareness of population explosion created, the birth rate tends to decrease and the death rate already having reached its lowest, the net resultant increase in population may be neutralised when the population tends to be stationary. This stage is known as *low stationary stage.*

v. With excessive use of birth control measures, the birth rate may fall below that of death rate as certain amount of deaths are imminent and death rate cannot be brought down below a certain level. At this stage the population may start declining. This stage is known as *declining stage.*

At present most of the developing and under developed countries are in the first three stages of population growth. Indian population was until recently in the early expanding stage and now is tending to step into late expanding stage.

Sources of Demographic Data

Demographic data required for monitoring of health activities mainly comprises of the estimates of population, births and deaths. These can be obtained from various sources. Some of the important sources are detailed below—

For population data

i. Census reports and Population estimates

For births

i. Registers of births
ii. Baptism records at churches

For deaths

i. Registers of deaths
ii. Registers at the burial and cremation ground
iii. Postmortem records

Population data sources are described in detail below.

Census Operations in India

This is the main source of data for population estimates. Census is a process of complete enumeration of all individuals in a country on a fixed date or period. In census, in addition to the counting of the total number of people, certain other information of importance are also collected. The information pertaining to the individuals such as age, sex, religion, caste, occupation, literacy, housing, income, etc. are also obtained at the time of census. Published census reports contain the information pertaining to the populations according to the above categorisation for each geographical area in the country in addition to the total population of each place at the time of census.

The first official census was undertaken in the World at Sweden in the year 1749. In India the first countrywide census took place in 1872, although the population census were conducted for individual areas prior to that date also. Subsequently census is taking place once in every ten years at the first year of each decade. The last census was in 2001 and the next one will be in 2011.

The scope and content of the Indian census has been expanding over the decades to cater to the needs of various Ministries of Government of India, Planning Commission, State Governments and other Institutions.

In 2001 census, information was collected using three schedules, the House list, the Household schedule and the Individual slip, pertaining to the period February-March, 2001.

The 'house list' contained information such as identification particulars of census houses, the use to which the houses are put to, the identification particulars of households, the members living in the census houses and particulars of physically handicapped persons in the households.

The 'household schedule' filled up for each household had two parts. The first part contained information relating to the household, including items such as household size, number of couples living in the household, amenities available in the household, household ownership of house/site, land and house hold cultivation. It also contained information on religion and information on scheduled caste/scheduled tribe, characteristics of head of household and language mainly spoken in the household. Part II of this schedule elicited information on the population record and had items such as list of members of the household, their socio-demographic and economic characteristics.

The third schedule which is the 'individual slip', contained two sets of information, one pertained to all the individuals, 'universal slip', while the other was only for population in 20% of the sampled rural and urban census blocks. This is the first time in the history of Indian census, that a few information was collected on a sample basis only.

The 'universal slip' used for collection of information on all the individuals, included particulars on demographic, social and cultural items including information on school attendance. These items covered the relationship to head of household, age, sex, marital status, religion, mother tongue other languages spoken, whether belonged to scheduled caste/ tribe, literacy, educational level and work status.

The information collected for sampled individuals were on migration and fertility status.

Some of the information published from the census data during 2001, census are contained in the following reports :

i. Primary census abstracts
ii. Final population totals
iii. Tables on houses, household amenities and assets
iv. General information
v. Scheduled castes
vi. Scheduled tribes
vii. Religious compositions
viii. Age-structures
ix. District population booklets
x. District population profiles
xi. Data on disability
xii. Population atlas

Besides the above series, some special papers are also being published. Some of these information are available on *Website* of Indian Census Directorate.

Definition of Terms Used in Indian Census

A thorough exercise on standardisation of questionnaires and the terms used therein were done before actual data collection through census. Some of the definitions of terms adopted at the 2001 census are given below. (Source : Census of India, 2001, H Series) (GOI).

i. *Rural Urban Classification*

For the purpose of census, urban areas have been so defined as to include:

a) All places with Municipal Corporation, Municipality, Notified Area Committee, Cantonment Board, etc.
b) All other places which satisfy the following criteria—
    - A minimum population of 5,000
    - At least 75 percent of the male working population being engaged in non agricultural pursuits and
    - Density of population of at least 400 persons per sq.m.

Places satisfying the above criteria are identified as Census towns or non-statutory towns by the Director of Census Operations, in each State and Union Territory.

Areas, which are neither notified by the State Government nor identified by the Director of Census Operations as urban or urban agglomeration, have been treated as rural.

ii. *Urban Agglomeration*

An urban agglomeration has been defined as out growths such as railway colonies, university campuses, port areas, military camps, etc. that have come up near a statutory town/ city but within the revenue limits of a village or villages contiguous to the town or city.

iii. *Occupied Residential Houses*

A census house is a building or a part of a building having a separate main entrance from the road or common courtyard or staircase, etc. used or recognised as a separate unit. It may be inhabited or vacant and may be used for residential or non-residential purposes or both. Occupied residential house means a census house, which is being used for residential purpose either partly or wholly.

iv. *Household*

A household is a group of persons who commonly live together and would take their meals from a common kitchen unless the exigencies of work prevented any of them from doing so. There may be a one member household, two member household or multi-member household. For census purposes each one of these types is regarded as a household. Again there may be a household of persons related by blood or household of unrelated persons, or having a mix of both. Examples of unrelated households are boarding houses, hostels, residential hotels or orphanages, rescue homes, ashrams, etc. These are called as *institutional households*. Again there may be household that does not have a house to live in. Such household may be itinerant in nature consisting of nomadic persons or living in such places which cannot be termed as houses.

v. *Literate*

A person who can both read and write with understanding in any language is treated as literate for the purpose of census. A person who can merely read but cannot write is not a literate. It is not necessary that a person, who is literate should have received any formal education or should have passed any minimum educational standard.

Population Estimation Methods

For the study of all indicators related to health, population is the basic one. As such it is essential to have a knowledge of the population of a country, a state or a district or even a community. Methods of population estimation for any area are given below.

The population of any area can be obtained either by the census report or through population estimates for inter-censal periods. Different methods of calculation of inter-censal population estimates are as follows.

i. *Natural Increase Method*

In this case the number of births, deaths, immigration and emigrations are taken into account for estimating the population during any year.

Thus estimated population at a period
= Population during the preceding Census
+ No. of (births – deaths) during the period after preceding census
+ No. of (immigrants – emigrants) during the period after the preceding census.

ii. *Arithmetical Progression Method*

In this method it is assumed that the population increase is in an arithmetic progression from year to year or between two census periods. In other words the rate of increase of population from one year to another is constant and is same from year to year between two census periods.

To estimate the population during any year, the rate of increase is calculated from the previous two census populations. This annual rate of increase is used in estimating the population at any time from the following formula:

$$P_t = P_0 + rt$$

where, P_t is the population at a period t years after the preceding census, r is the annual rate of increase of population which is obtained as (1/10) of the difference between the population estimates at the previous two successive census and P_0 is the population estimate at the immediate preceding census.

Example 14.1. The calculation of population estimate of Bangalore Urban Agglomeration (U.A.) for the year 2007 by the above method is illustrated below.

Population of Bangalore UA in 1991 : 4,130,288
Population of Bangalore UA in 2001 : 5,686,844
Population increase in 10 years = 1556556

Increase for one year = 155656

Increase in population for 6 years from 2001 to 2007, Census reference period

= (155656 x 6) = 933936

Population of Bangalore UA on Census reference period of 2007

= (5,686,844 + 933936)

= 6,620,780

Similarly population estimate at any reference period can be calculated, taking the duration from the previous Census period.

iii. *Geometric Progression Method*

In this method, it is assumed that the population increase from year to year will be in a geometric progression or in other words the population increases from year to year in a constant ratio.

To estimate the population by this method, the constant ratio of increase is obtained from the previous two census population estimates using geometric increase method, which will be geometric growth rate and the population estimate at any period is obtained from the formula.

$$P_t = P_0 (1 + r)^t$$

Where P_t is the estimated population at a period t after previous Census.

P_0 is the population estimate at the previous census.

r is the annual geometric growth rate of population between the two census periods, obtained from the population estimates at the previous two census.

The estimation of population by this method is illustrated in the following example.

Example 14.2. To estimate the population of Bangalore UA for the year 2007, for the data given in Example 14.1,

First the annual growth rate is calculated as follows—

P_0 = Population of Bangalore U.A. in 1991 = 4,130,288

P_t = Population of Bangalore U.A. in 2001 = 5,686,844

t = Number of years between the two Census = 10

Substituting these values in the above equation, $P_t = P_0 (1+ r)^t$ and taking logarithms to base 10, of both sides,

$$\log P_t = \log P_0 + t \log (1 + r)$$

$$\text{or} \quad \log (1 + r) = (1/10) (\log P_t - \log P_0)$$

$$= (1/10) (\log 5{,}686{,}844 - \log 4{,}130{,}288)$$

$$= (1/10) (6.754871 - 6.615980)$$

$$= (1/10) (0.138891)$$

$$= 0.0138891$$

$$(1+r) = \text{Antilog } (0.0138891)$$

$$= 1.0325$$

$$r = (1.0325 - 1) = 0.0325$$

Substituting this geometric growth rate of population,

Population of Bangalore UA at 2007 reference period of census is estimated as

$P_t = 5{,}686{,}844 (1 + 0.0325)^6$, since t is 6 years after previous census.

Taking logarithms to base 10, on both sides,

$$\log (\text{Population at } 2007) = \log (5{,}686{,}844) + 6 \log (1.0325)$$

$$= 6.754871 + 0.083340 = 6.838211$$

Population of Bangalore U.A. at 2007 = Antilog (6.838211)

= 6,889,870

iv. *Other Methods of Population Projection*

It can be seen that the above two methods have assumed that the population growth rate as existed between the two previous census period has not changed from year to year. But there will be continuous changes in migration status, fertility patterns, etc. which influence population growth rates. As such population estimations are now being made with various assumptions and with different mathematical models, taking these changes into consideration.

Vital Statistics Registration

a. *Channel of Registration of Vital Statistics*

Records of births and deaths are fundamental necessities of health statistics as they are most helpful in working out indices like birth and death rates, causes of deaths, population projections, planning of health services or assessing the progress of health measures undertaken. Registration of births and deaths were recognised long before 1250 BC in Egypt. Churches started maintaining the records of baptisms, marriages and deaths. However, Sweden and Finland were the first countries to make these registrations as a civilian affair and they were used for calculation of vital statistical indices. In various other countries like Europe and America the system of registration developed only in 18th and 19th centuries. By 1933 the registration laws covered about half of World's population and by 1955 it was about 60%.

In India, before independence, in some states, the registration of births and deaths were not compulsory. After the dawn of independence in India, even though, these registrations were compulsory in every state, the laws pertaining to them varied from State to State and were not uniform. However, an act of parliament was enforced for the compulsory registration of births and deaths, through out the country and this has come into force from April, 1970.

The channel of compilation of births and deaths are slightly different in urban and rural areas and are as follows:

In *urban areas* such as municipalities, cantonments, notified areas and corporations, the whole locality is divided into certain number of wards and Ward Registrars maintain these records in each ward. Heads of the families in which a birth or death occurs are bound by obligation of law to report, any birth or death occurring in their families, to these Ward Registrars, within seven days for births and three days for deaths from the occurrence of the event. In bigger towns there are registration offices at the burial and burning *ghats* and they keep the record of deaths. Heads of hospitals, *Dharmasalas* and maternity homes should also report the events to the Ward Registrars. To avoid omissions sweepers, midwives and dais have to report every occurrence that comes to their knowledge. Ward Registrars send the returns, once in a week, to the Municipal Health Officer and in the absence of such health officer to the Executive Officer of the Municipality.

Returns are sent direct to the state Directors of Health by the Municipal Medical Officer of health once a month.

In *rural areas* the primary unit of registration of births and deaths is the *Gram Panchayat*. The *Panchayat* secretary maintains the birth and death registers. Reports are sent to the Block Development Officer at the Block level. From here the returns are sent to the State Director of Medical and Health Services once a month. This state level return is then sent to the Registrar General of Vital Statistics attached to the Director General of Health Services at the National level where the returns are compiled for the whole country.

The international level report is compiled by the World Health Organisation at Geneva.

The Registrar General of Vital Statistics at the National level and the State Directors of Medical and Health Services at the State Level publish these data once a year.

b. *Lapses in the Registration System of Vital Statistics*

In India, only in 1970 a uniform law for the registration of births and deaths have come into force. Previous to this period the laws were not uniform from state to state. The under-registration of births and deaths ranged up to 80%.

The situation was almost similar in rural as well as in urban areas. The causes for this under registration are as follows:-

i. Both in rural and urban areas the primary responsibility of reporting of events rests with the head of the family where the event has occurred. With high illiteracy rate prevailing in the country, the public are not conscious of the importance of these statistics and as such most of the times they never report the statistics.
ii. Even though the laws exist for imposing punishment for non-reporting, the laws are rarely enforced.
iii. In rural areas the *Gram Panchayat* Chairman and the *Panchayat* secretary who are primarily responsible for maintenance of these records, are multifarious workers and they never give much importance for maintaining these records. Further they are not employees of the health department.
iv. The death records, which are the main source of information of age at death as well as the cause of death, are never complete. The age and the cause of death are seldom recorded correctly.
v. There is a time lag in the compilation and transmission of these statistics from one agency to the other in the channel of compilation, as such the statistics at the higher levels are mostly under compiled.

Thus the coverage of vital statistics registration is defective both quantitatively and qualitatively.

Schemes for the Improvement of Vital Statistics Registration System

Various schemes have been implemented in recent years to improve the quality and quantity of vital statistics. Both long term and short-term schemes have been in operation, to get quick and reliable estimates of vital statistics and also statistics relating to the causes of death. The two important schemes in this direction are outlined below.

i. *Sample Registration Scheme (SRS)*

This scheme is implemented to provide reliable estimates of birth rates, death rates and other fertility indicators at both State level as well as at all India level, separately for rural and urban areas. The scheme was initiated by the Office of the Registrar General of India on a pilot basis in 1964-65 and became fully operational in 1969-70, in about 3700 sample units. At present, the scheme is operational in 4436 rural units and 2235 urban units. A rural unit comprises of a village or a segment of a village with about 1500 population while an urban unit comprises of a census enumeration block with a population ranging from 750 to 1000. These units are selected on random sample basis with in each State. Local residents like teachers, midwives, village level worker, etc. are appointed as part time enumerators and are given intensive training. They are paid monthly honorarium. These enumerators maintain a layout map of their respective areas. The population base is collected on a household schedule. They also maintain a list of pregnant women. Every birth or death is recorded as and when they occur. This information is collected through reliable informants like barber, village *dai*, washerman, village priest, etc. These events are recorded by the enumerator only after satisfying himself of the occurrence of the event.

A half-yearly survey-cum-enumeration is also carried out by the supervisor and the lists prepared by the enumerator and the supervisor are matched. Unmatched events in the two lists are verified jointly by them or by a third person. The final lists are transmitted to the Registrar General of India, where the countrywide statements are prepared.

Thus SRS has the unique feature of recording the vital events both in a longitudinal manner as well as through a periodical survey. The longitudinal method of recording avoids the bias inherent in recall lapse. The events are recorded on *de jure* basis and proper accounting of these events according to permanent residents and visitors are also done.

Sample Registration System information is published periodically through their Bulletin by Registrar General of India.

ii. *Model Registration*

The scheme mainly envisages collection of data on causes of deaths by para-medical staff. For this purpose, certain Primary health centres are provided with field agents who are assigned some area of work. These field agents contact local informants regularly at short intervals and collect the addresses of the dead persons. Then each of these field agents visits these households in his area and obtains necessary information and ensures that the event has occurred within the village and not outside, irrespective of the fact that the event pertains to a person resident of the village or not. He assigns a probable cause of death. He also collects information about births in the village so as to keep watch over infant deaths and deaths due to childbirth and complication of pregnancy. For assigning the cause of death he consults the Manual of Instruction provided to him. At the end of each month the field agent is required to prepare a report and send it to the Recorder at Primary health centre who after scrutinising submits it to the Medical Officer for checking and onward transmission to the state headquarters. The monthly returns received at the State headquarters are compiled and a consolidated statement is sent to the Registrar General of India for further checking, processing and analysis.

At the end of half year, i.e. 30th June and 31st December of every year the field agents rechecks occurrence of any death or birth by house to house enquiry and matches with similar information collected during continuous recording. The events recorded wrongly are deleted. The Medical Officer of the Primary Health Centre is also expected to check ten percent of the deaths reported by the field agent. Thus the model registration aims more at quantitative rather than qualitative assessment of mortality pattern. Number of Primary Health Centres selected for this scheme is approximately equal to the quotient obtained by dividing the population by one lakh.

15 Chapter Health Indicators

Importance of Health Indicators

It is the primary need of any health administrator to have some indices of measurement of health status in his community. These are required not only to help him in his task of efficiently maintaining the health of the community but also in assessing the specific problems, for planning his service programmes in an efficient manner and also in evaluating his programmes. These indicators will also enable him to compare the health status of different areas as well as to compare the health status of an area over a period of time. There are various indicators designed for these purposes and they are known as Health indicators. Nature of these indicators vary according to their utility. For calculating these indicators, the data should be collected accurately and from reliable sources as well as from large number of observations.

Concept of Measures of Health

It is known that the best estimate to express a series of quantitative observations in a concise manner is the mean or the average. But for all qualitative observations involving attributes, a similar estimate would be a ratio.

A ratio can be defined as an index giving the relative magnitude of one character in terms of the other. For example, the ratio of Tuberculosis cases in India during the year 1995 was 47:10,000. This means that for every 10,000 persons there were 47 cases of Tuberculosis in India. Similarly the number of females for every 1000 males can be expressed as Sex ratio. In Karnataka State, during 2001 census, the sex ratio was 963:1000, which means that the number of females for every 1000 males in the State was 963.

Generally, Ratios when expressed for a particular base, for a definite interval of time and geographical area, are known as rates. The base usually chosen for health indicator is either 100 or 1000 and the interval of time will be a calendar year, a month, a fortnight or a week as per situations.

In rates, the numerator gives the number of times certain event has happened while the denominator gives the number of times there was an exposure to the event.

From the above criteria, it can be observed that a rate gives the probability of an event to happen and also from these probabilities one can calculate the expected number of such events in a population by multiplying the probability by the total population of the area.

A few examples of these rates are birth rate, death rate, infant mortality rate, morbidity rates, fertility rates etc. which are discussed in detail in the subsequent paragraphs.

Types of Health Indicators

Health indicators can be grouped under five broad areas:

i. Demographic indicators
ii. Morbidity indicators
iii. Mortality indicators
iv. Health service indicators
v. Hospital management indicators

Each of the above indicators has its own applicability and use in a particular type of situation. For calculation of these indicators, accurate data is necessary in terms of the population exposed for a particular event as well as the number of events in an area over a period of time. Details and calculation formulae for important indicators are provided below.

Demographic Indicators

a. *Population of an Area*

For the study of all other indicators, population is the basic one. Population of any area during a particular period can be obtained either by census estimates, or population projection methods already described or through specific surveys.

b. *Crude Birth Rate*

This rate indicates the number of live births taking place during a year in a community for every 1000 persons living in the community.

This is calculated as

Crude birth rate =

$$\frac{\text{(No. of live births registered or estimated during a year in an area)} \times 1000}{\text{(Mid-year estimate of the total population of the area)}}$$

Example 15.1. In a sample survey of a Community Development Block with an estimated population of 9832 during a year, the number of live births reported were 343.

$$\text{Crude birth rate in the area} = \frac{343 \times 1000}{9832}$$

$$= 34.9$$

This rate is useful for assessing the trends in the number of births occurring from year to year in the population, for estimating the total population at any time and for assessing the fertility status of a community.

But the crude birth rate has its own limitations. As the population consists of various age groups of men and women of both child bearing and non-child bearing age groups, this rate does not take into account the differences in the fertility pattern of the community.

c. *General Fertility Rate*

A refined estimate of the fertility would be the General fertility rate which is the number of live births in a year in an area for every 1000 women in reproductive age group, i.e.,15-44 years.

This is calculated as :

General fertility rate

$$= \frac{\text{(No. of live births registered or estimated in an area during a year)} \times 1000}{\text{(No. of estimated women aged 15-44 years in the area during the year)}}$$

Example 15.2. In the survey data referred above, number of females in the age group 15-44 years were 1788 and the number of live births reported by them during the year were 343.

$$\text{General fertility rate of the area} = \frac{343 \times 1000}{1788}$$

$$= 191.8$$

Fertility rates are useful in comparing fertility trends from year to year, as a measure of the effectiveness of the family planning programmes.

d. *Age Specific Fertility Rate*

Instead of calculating the fertility rates for the entire age group 15-44 years, they can be calculated for specific age groups also. Such rates are known as age-specific fertility rates. As an example age specific fertility rate for any age group can be calculated as :

Age Specific Fertility Rate for any age group =

$$\frac{\text{(No. of live births reported by mothers in a particular age group in an area during the year)} \times 1000}{\text{(Estimated number of mothers in the particular age group in the area during the year)}}$$

Example 15.3. In the survey data referred above, number of live births reported by 751 mothers in the age group 15-24 were 131.

Age specific fertility rate for the age group 15 to 24

$$= \frac{131 \times 1000}{751}$$

$$= 174.4$$

e. *Total Fertility Rate*

This is an estimate of the average number of children that would be born to a woman if she experiences the current fertility pattern throughout her reproductive span of life of

15 to 44 years. This is obtained as a sum of all the single year age specific fertility rates for all the years of reproductive span of life. When five-year age specific fertility rates are considered the total is to be multiplied by 5 to get the total fertility rate. This rate gives an idea as to how many children would be born to a women, during her entire span of reproductive life under the existing fertility conditions.

f. *Age Specific Marital Fertility Rate*

Since the general fertility rate does not take into account the marital status of women in the any age group, a refined estimate of the fertility rate can be obtained as the number of live births in a year per thousand married women in any specified age group.

g. *Gross Reproduction Rate*

In the calculation of this rate only female births are considered as they are going to be the potential mothers. As such this rate is expressed as the average number of daughters that would be born to a woman if she experiences the current fertility pattern throughout her reproductive span of life,15 to 44 years. Calculation of this rate is done similar to that of total fertility rate but only female births are taken into consideration instead of all births.

h. *Net Reproduction Rate*

In the calculation of gross reproduction rate, no consideration was given for the mortality of mothers in various age groups. After correcting for the mortality of mothers in various age groups, net reproduction rate is calculated as the number of female children that would be born on an average to a woman under prevailing mortality and fertility considerations.

Morbidity Indicators

Before discussing different morbidity indicators, understanding of the following basic concepts of measurement of morbidity are necessary.

In a broad sense, morbidity may be defined as any departure, subjective or objective from a state of well being resulting from a disease, an injury or an impairment. This can be further amplified keeping the meaning of well being from WHO definition of Health as a '"State of complete physical, mental and social well being and not merely an absence of disease or infirmity".

The morbidity may be prevailing already at the time of commencement of an investigation or may commence during the period of observation.

As such basic data required for the calculation of morbidity indicators are:

(i) Number of persons ill at any time,
(ii) Number of episodes of sickness starting during a period,
(iii) Number of spells or attacks of the disease,
(iv) Duration of the illness,
(v) Number of deaths from the disease.

Important morbidity indicators and their calculation procedures are detailed below.

a. *Incidence Rate*

This rate provides an idea about the new cases of any sickness that occur during a period for 1000 population in an area and is calculated as:

Incidence rate of any disease

$$= \frac{\text{(No. of cases of the disease that occur during a period in an year)} \times 1000}{\text{(Average number of persons exposed to the risk during the period in the area)}}$$

This rate can be calculated for the number of cases of a sickness or spells of that sickness.

Average number of persons exposed to risk is the average of the estimated population of the area at the beginning and end of the period of consideration and if this period is an year, it will be midyear population estimate of the area for that year.

Example 15.4. During the year of survey in the example referred previously, the number of GIT disease cases which occurred during the year were 208 out of the population of 9832.

Incidence rate of GIT diseases for the year

$$= \frac{(208 \times 1000)}{9832}$$

$$= 21.1 \text{ per } 1000 \text{ population.}$$

b. *Prevalence Rate*

This is an indicator which provides information about the quantum of any sickness that is present during an interval of time or at a point of time for 1000 population in an area.

If it is expressed for an interval of time, it is called as Period prevalence rate and if it is for a point of time it will be called a Point prevalence rate.

They are calculated as follows :

Period prevalence rate of any disease =

$$\frac{\text{(No. of cases of any disease present during a period in an area)} \times 1000}{\text{(Average number of persons exposed to the risk of the disease during the period in the area)}}$$

Point prevalence rate of any disease =

$$\frac{\text{(No. of cases a disease existing at the point of time in an area) x 1000}}{\text{(No. of persons exposed to the risk of the disease at that point of time in the area)}}$$

Example 15.5. In the survey referred above, number of filariasis disease cases detected at the time of survey were 80 out of a population of 11970 surveyed for the disease.

Point prevalence rate of filariasis for the area

$$= \frac{80 \times 1000}{11970}$$

$$= 6.68 \text{ per } 1000 \text{ population}$$

c. *Case Fatality Rate*

It gives the extent of fatality of any disease and is expressed as the number of deaths of persons due to a particular disease for every 1000 cases or attacks of that disease during a period in the area.

It is calculated as :

Case fatality rate of a disease =

$$\frac{\text{(No. of death reported from a specific disease during a period in an area)} \times 1000}{\text{(No. of cases reported of the specific disease during the period in the area)}}$$

Example 15.6. In the survey referred above, the number of deaths reported due to GIT diseases were 31 out of the total number of 208 cases. The Case fatality rate due to GIT diseases is calculated as follows—

Case fatality rate due to GIT diseases in the area

$$= \frac{(31 \times 1000)}{208}$$

$$= 149.0 \text{ per } 1000 \text{ cases}$$

Mortality Indicators

These are the indicators which are useful in understanding the extent of total mortality or deaths due to various causes in an area. Various indicators in terms of age groups, causes etc. are calculated. Important mortality indicators are detailed below.

a. *Crude Death Rate*

The extent of deaths taking place in the area due to all causes and in all age groups is expressed by crude death rate. This is defined as the number of deaths occurring per thousand population in an area during a year.

It is calculated from the formula :

Crude death rate =

$$\frac{\text{(No. of deaths registered or estimated during a year in an area)} \times 1000}{\text{(Mid year estimated population of the area)}}$$

Example 15.7. In the survey referred above, the total number of deaths were 125 out of an estimated population of 9832. Crude death rate of the area

$$= \frac{(125 \times 1000)}{9832}$$

$$= 12.7$$

The crude death rate provides an overall picture about the deaths in an area but will not indicate any other details such as the deaths according to the causes, age groups or sex groups. Mortality conditions in several age groups vary in earlier and later age groups of life. Deaths are more common in the early age groups, while they are lesser in the middle age groups. Further males and females do not have same mortality conditions. As such crude death rate is a summary of mortality conditions in an area.

b. *Age and Sex Specific Death Rate*

In order to estimate the extent of deaths in various age groups and according to age and sex and age and sex specific death rates are useful. This is defined as the number of deaths in any age group of a particular sex, per thousand population of that particular age and sex group during a year in an area.

It is calculated as :

Age and sex specific death rate for any age and sex group

$$= \frac{\text{(No. of deaths registered or estimated in an age and sex group during a year in an area)} \times 1000}{\text{(Estimated population of that age and sex group for the period in the area)}}$$

Example 15.8. In the community survey mentioned above, out of the total deaths, the number of male deaths in the age group 1 to 4 years were 31, out of a population of 1152 in that age and sex group.

Age and sex specific death rate for 1 to 4 years for males

$$= \frac{(31 \times 1000)}{1152}$$

$$= 26.9$$

c. *Infant Mortality Rate*

This is an indicator which estimates the death of children in the first year of life and is defined as the number of deaths of children before completing one year of age for every 1000 children below the age of one year. But it is difficult to get the exact number of children in the first year of life, as such usually the number of live births recorded during the year is taken as an approximate estimate of the children below one year of age.

It is calculated as :

Infant mortality rate (IMR) =

$$\frac{\text{(No. of deaths registered or estimated of children below one year during a year in an area)} \times 1000}{\text{No. of live births, registered or estimated during the year in the area}}$$

It may be noted that Infant mortality rate (IMR) is actually the age specific death rate during the first year of life. One of the major causes of deaths of infants in our country are diarrhoeas and dysentries which are caused due to bad environmental sanitation. As such the infant mortality rate is considered as an index of environmental sanitation conditions of an area.

Example 15.9. In the survey mentioned above the estimated number of deaths of infants during the year was 47 and the corresponding number of live births was 343.

$$\text{IMR} = \frac{(47 \times 1000)}{343}$$
$$= 137.0$$

d. *Neonatal Mortality Rate*

As a further sub-division of infant mortality, the number of deaths of children below one year can be analysed according to age groups. When only the deaths under 28 days of age are considered, Neonatal mortality rate can be calculated as the number of deaths of children below the age of 28 days for every 1000 live births in the area during the year under consideration. This rate provides an estimate of the deaths due to causes of endogenous factors such as birth injuries, neonatal tetanus and congenital disorders. Nearly 45 percent of the total deaths below 1 year occur during this age period.

This rate is calculated as :

Neonatal mortality rate

$$= \frac{\text{(No. of deaths registered or estimated of children below 28 days of age during a year} \times 1000}{\text{(No. of live births registered or estimated during the year in the area)}}$$

e. *Postneonatal Mortality Rate*

This rate provides us an estimate of the infant deaths after 28 days of life for every 1000 live births in the area. In India major causes of deaths in this age group are due to bad environmental sanitation, malnutrition and infections. As such this rate provides an estimate of such conditions prevailing in the community.

This rate is calculated as :

Postneonatal mortality rate =

$$\frac{\text{(No. of deaths registered or estimated of infants above 28 days of age in an area during a year)} \times 1000}{\text{(No. of estimated live births in the area during the year)}}$$

f. *Perinatal Mortality Rate*

This rate takes into account the number of late foetal deaths (still births) and deaths during very early stages of infancy i.e. up to one week of life.

This rate is calculated as :

Perinatal mortality rate

$$= \frac{\text{(Late foetal deaths (28 weeks or more) + No. of deaths under one week in an area during a year)} \times 1000}{\text{(Estimated number of (live birth +still births) in the area during the year)}}$$

This provides us a sensitive indicator reflecting the standards, availability and utilisation of Obstetrics as well as Paediatric services in an area.

g. *Disease Specific Death Rate*

This rate reflects the mortality condition in an area according to a cause group. This will be useful in knowing the extent of major causes of mortality in the population to plan suitable measures to reduce the mortality due to these causes. This indicator is defined as the number of deaths due to a specific cause or disease during the year for one thousand population in the area.

It is calculated as :

Disease specific death rate for any disease =

$$\frac{\text{(No. of deaths registered or estimated during a year due to a specific disease in the area)} \times 1000}{\text{(Mid year or estimated population of the area during the year)}}$$

Example 15.10. In the survey referred above, during the year, out of an estimated population of 9832, 31 deaths due to GIT diseases were reported.

Disease specific death rate due to GIT diseases for the area during the year

$$= \frac{(31 \times 1000)}{9832}$$
$$= 3.2 \text{ per 1000 population}$$

h. *Maternal Mortality Rate*

This indicator provides information on the extent of deaths of mothers due to pregnancy and puerperal causes and is defined as the number of deaths of females due to pregnancy, and complications of pregnancy for every 1000 births during the year.

It is calculated as :

Maternal mortality rate =

$$\frac{\text{(No. of female deaths registered or estimated during a year due to pregnancy or its complications in an area)} \times 1000}{\text{(No. of registered or estimated live births during the year in the area)}}$$

Example 15.11. In the survey referred above, 3 maternal deaths and 343 live births were reported.

Maternal mortality rate during the year for the area

$$= \frac{(3 \times 1000)}{343} = 8.75$$

i. *Proportional Mortality Ratio*

This indicator is used to know the percentage of deaths after a certain age. This has been defined as the percentage of deaths at the age of 50 and over for the total deaths in an area.

This is calculated as :

Proportional Mortality Ratio =

$$\frac{\text{(Number of deaths of people of age 50 and over in an area during a year)} \times 100}{\text{(Total number of deaths of all ages in the area during the year)}}$$

This index would be 100 if all persons survive up to an age of 50 years while it would be zero if no one reaches the age of 50.

j. *Expectation of Life*

This is an indicator used to give an idea about the average duration of life in years at a certain age in an area, calculated from the Life tables. Expectation of life calculated at birth gives the average number of years a newborn is expected to survive. It can be calculated for different ages also.

Indicators of Health Services

Even though health services are available, many of them are not reaching the population. As such WHO. Expert Committees on health indicators have suggested some indicators for the measurement of the availability and extent of usage of health services. Some of these are listed as follows—

a. *Environmental health indicators*

i. Percentage of population in a community receiving protected water supply,
ii. Percentage of population in a community having facilities for proper disposal of excreta.

b. *Medical care indicators*

i. Availability of medical and paramedical personnel per thousand population in a community,
ii. Availability and extent of usage of various medical facilities like dispensaries, hospitals etc. per thousand population in a community.

Hospital Management Indicators

Indicators, which are helpful in the assessment of performance of a hospital, are outlined below with the formula for their calculation.

i. Bed Turnover Rate (BTR) indicates the number of patients who have been given services per bed year. It is calculated as:

$$BTR = \frac{\text{Total number of discharges during the year} \times 100}{\text{Total number of authorised beds}}$$

ii. Bed Occupancy Rate (BOR) is the ratio of occupied bed days to the available bed days as determined by bed capacity, during any given period. It is calculated as :

$$\text{BOR} = \frac{\text{Actual number of occupied bed days} \times 100}{\text{Available bed days}}$$

iii. Length of stay of patients provides an estimate of the average period of stay of patients in a ward and is calculated as an average number of days stayed by all the patients in a given period of time.

Chapter 16 Standardisation of Rates

Meaning and Need for Standardisation

Comparison of various rates concerning human populations either of different groups or of the same group over a period of time requires a careful thinking. The fact that one place has a higher crude death rate or a disease specific morbidity rate as compared to another does not necessarily mean that the conditions of general mortality or the prevalence of a particular disease in the place with higher rates is worse than the other. It is well known that the mortality conditions as well as the incidence of most of the diseases vary from one age group to the other as well as between the sexes. It is quite evident that the age specific death rates in lower age groups and upper age groups are higher as compared to middle age groups. As an example, when observations are made in a community with higher proportions of middle aged people and compared with a community with large proportions of other age groups, it is obvious that the crude death rate of the former would be less than the crude death rate of the latter. This difference in the crude death rate between the two communities may be mainly due to the differences in the age structure of the two communities and may not be because of the differences in the mortality conditions in the area. Similarly in addition to age structure, the sex structure will also play a role in bringing about the differences in the crude death rate between the communities.

Hence, in order to compare either the mortality conditions or the disease conditions between places or over a period of time, the over all rates for the area are to be standardised with reference to age and sex groups and then comparisons are to be made. That is to say that the over all rates for the communities are to be calculated after giving due weights and standardised for the age and sex structure of the community as well as the age and sex specific rates of the event under study. Then only the over all comparisons will yield a correct picture. Two methods of standardisation of overall rates are discussed below.

Direct Method of Standardisation (Table 16.1)

In this method an estimate of the total expected events in the community of either the number of cases of a specific disease under study or the number of deaths is obtained by applying the age and sex specific rates of the event for the community under study to the age and sex structure of a standard population. On the basis of this total number of events, the over all rate for the community is calculated which is called as the standardised rate of the events for the community. Utilising such standardised rates calculated for different communities, comparisons can be made between them. Usually the standard population chosen will be that of the age and sex structure of the whole country reduced to one million population. In the absence of this standard million, any other suitable age and sex structure applicable to the communities under comparisons can be utilised. Thus in this method, standardised rates are calculated by estimating the events for a common age and sex structure, whereby the effect of the differences in the age and sex composition of the communities under comparison is eliminated. In other words, in this method of standardisation the events in the community are estimated as if the age and sex structure of the standard population is exposed to the conditions prevailing in the community.

The method of calculating standardised rate by the direct method is illustrated in the following example:

Example 16.1. In a community the stool positivity rates between two sections of a community is compared in terms of over all percentage infestation rates. This rate for the two sections of the community is standardised by direct method by applying the age specific infestation rates to the age structure of the total population of the community. Thus in this case the age structure of the community as a whole has been taken as the standard population.

The different values in the columns of the table are obtained as follows.

In column 1, the age groups for which age specific rates are available are entered.

In columns (2) and (3), the age specific rates for the two groups are entered.

In column (4), the standard population age structure is taken. Columns (5) and (6) contain the estimated number of events which are obtained by multiplying the age specific rate of the groups and the respective standard population in that age group.

Standardised rate

$$= \frac{\text{(No. of estimated events for a community)} \times 100}{\text{Total population of the community}}$$

Standardised percentage stool positivity amongst middle socio-economic group

$$= \frac{1248.3 \times 100}{3069}$$

$$= 40.7$$

Standardised percentage stool positivity amongst lower socio-economic group

$$= \frac{1360.8 \times 100}{3069}$$

$$= 44.4$$

Indirect Method of Standardisation

Direct method of standardisation requires the knowledge of age specific rates of the events under comparison for each of the communities as well as the standard population age structure. Sometimes, the above data may not be available or the population in different age or sex groups or may be too small resulting in large fluctuations of the age specific rates

Table 16.1: Calculation of standardised rate by direct method

Age group in years	Percentage stool positives		Total population of the area taken as standard population	Estimated number of stool positives in the Standard population	
	Middle Socio-economic-group	Lower socio-economic group		As per middle socio-economic group rates	As per lower socio-economic group rates
(1)	(2)	(3)	(4)	(5)	(6)
0-5	52.2	55.7	505	263.6	281.3
6-10	38.1	58.1	448	170.7	260.3
11-20	52.6	45.6	669	351.9	305.1
21-30	24.1	39.7	554	133.5	219.9
31-40	29.4	34.1	400	117.6	136.4
Over 40	42.8	32.0	493	211.0	157.8
Total	**30.8**	**45.1**	**3069**	**1248.3**	**1360.8**

through the presence of only a few events. In such circumstances it is desirable to standardise the over all rates of each community by Indirect method of standardisation.

Indirect method of standardisation requires the knowledge of the age and sex structure of the population of each of the communities as well as the age and sex specific rates of events under consideration for the Standard population.

In this method of standardisation, first the number of events that would be expected if the local community is exposed to the age and sex specific rates of the events in the standard population is estimated. This is calculated by multiplying the age and sex specific rates of the Standard population and the population of the community in the corresponding age and sex groups. These estimates are summed up for the entire community and is then divided by the total population of the community and a rate is calculated for a suitable base. This rate is known as *Index Rate*. This index rate would show as to what would have been the over all rate for the community if it had the same conditions as prevailed in the standard population. This rate will be exactly equal to that of the standard population if the age and sex structure of the community would have been the same as that of Standard population. If it is different, then the observed over all rate for the community has to be adjusted by increasing or diminishing according to the situation. The quantity by which this adjustment is to be done is indicated by the ratio of the observed over all rate of the Standard population to the index rate of the community. This ratio is known as *Standardising Factor*.

The overall rate of the event for the community is multiplied by the Standardising factor to get the standardised rate for the community.

Thus the steps involved in this method of standardisation are as follows.

i. Calculate the index rate for community from the formula:

$$\text{Index rate} = \frac{\text{(Total number of estimated events for the community obtained by applying the age and sex specific rates of the Standard population to the age and sex structure of the community)} \times 1000}{\text{Total population of the community}}$$

The numerator is obtained by summing up the estimated events for each age and sex group which is obtained by multiplying the population in each age and sex group of the community with the corresponding age and sex specific rate of the event in the standard population.

ii. Calculate the standardising factor from the formula:
Standardising factor =

$$\frac{\text{Overall rate for the Standard population}}{\text{Index rate for the Community}}$$

iii. Calculate the standardised rate for the community as (Observed rate for the community) x (Standardising factor)

Example 16.2. The mortality data obtained by a sample survey of a community development block is given in the example for which the indirect method of standardisation is applied to obtain standardised death rate (Table 16.2) for the area.

Estimated number of deaths for each age and sex group is obtained by multiplying the population in that group by the corresponding age and sex specific death rates of rural India as in Table 16.2.

Table 16.2: Calculation of standardised death rate

Age in years	Population from a Community development block		Age and sex specific death rates of rural India for the year of study		Estimated no. of deaths for the sample	
	Males	Females	Males	Females	Males	Females
0 – 4	734	685	58.3	70.2	42.8	48.1
5 – 14	1494	1311	4.5	5.3	6.7	6.9
15 – 19	471	352	2.1	4.,2	1.0	1.5
20 – 24	397	399	3.9	5.5	1.5	2.2
25 - 29	386	362	3.7	5.5	1.4	2.0
30 – 34	339	327	4.1	6.4	1.4	2.1
35 – 39	293	239	6.5	6.1	1.9	1.5
40 – 44	260	206	8.5	7.6	2.2	1.6
45 – 49	187	170	13.2	9.4	2.5	1.6
50 – 54	187	168	18.7	16.2	3.5	2.7
55+	480	385	60.2	56.9	28.9	21.9
Total	5228	4604			93.8	92.1
Crude Death rate		12.7	19.1			

Total no. of estimated deaths in the sample population after applying standard population rates $= (93.8 + 92.1) = 185.9$

Index death rate for the community $= \dfrac{(185.9)\,(1000)}{9832}$

$= 18.91$

Standardising factor $= \dfrac{19.1}{18.91} = 1.01$

Standardised death rate for the community

$= 12.7 \times 1.01 = 12.8$

Here we can see that the standardised death rate of the area is not much different from the crude death rate of the area as the age and sex structure of the area is almost same as that of the Standard population i.e., Rural India.

Further it indicates that the mortality conditions in the Community Development Block is below that of the overall rural Indian population, as the Standardised Death rate in the Community under consideration which is 12.8 is below that of the Rural population of India as a whole which is 19.1.

17 Chapter

The Life Table

Concept of Life Table

The life table is the presentation of the mortality experience of a community during a given period. This table explains the mortality outcome of a specified population say 100,000 babies born at the same time, in terms of the number of people surviving up to different ages and also the average longevity of persons surviving up to an age. These tables were originally intended for the study of mortality experience as observed at the time of construction of the life table. But at present the life table technique is utilised for studying the incidence and outcome of populations exposed to certain chronic diseases and various other longitudinal studies.

Usually while constructing a standard life table, the group is started with a standard number like 100,000 or 1000 etc. born on a day or exposed to an event at a time. While studying mortality experience, this group gradually loses a certain number of members at each age according to a schedule that is fixed in advance as per the mortality conditions at each age. Further, the group will not change with reference to its membership except due to reduction because of death. It is also assumed that the deaths or the events under study are evenly distributed between one birthday and the next or between subsequent intervals under study. This group is usually constituted by members of the same sex.

The group with which the life table calculations are started and which is observed at different age periods is known as the Radix of the table.

The Radix of the life table gradually decreases when a study is made on the mortality experience of a community and it can be seen that the reduction is high in the early years of life and gradually decreases with the increase in the age till the middle age is reached and then again this reduction increases in the later years of life.

When the life table technique is used for the study of certain chronic diseases, the pattern may be different according to the age specific incidence and death rates.

Description of the Life Table

There are different rows and columns in a life table. Each row refers to some particular age x_i. This age is the exact number of completed years since birth.

As can be seen from the Table 17.1, the first column gives this age x and all other columns correspond to this age.

The second column l_x gives the number of persons who survive to exact age x out of the l_0 number of persons started at age 0.

The column q_x gives the probability that a person at exact age x will die before reaching the age (x + 1).

In some life tables there will be an additional column p_x which gives $(1 - q_x)$ as the probability that a person of age x will survive till he reaches the age (x + 1).

The column L_x gives the number of persons living between the ages x and (x + 1).

This is calculated approximately as

$$L_x = (l_x + l_{x+1}) / 2$$

This approximation is valid only when the deaths are evenly distributed between the years x and (x + 1).

The columns T_x gives the total number of years lived beyond x years by the L_x number of persons, reaching the age x.

This is obtained by adding to L_x, all the other values in this column beyond x years.

i.e., $T_x = L_x + L_{x+1} + L_{x+2}$ ....till all have died.

The column e^0_x gives the average number of years lived after age x by each of the l_x persons who attain that age.

This quantity is called as the *Expectation of life at age x.*

This is obtained as $e^0_x = \frac{T_x}{l_x}$

Thus e^0_x, gives the average number of years lived by the l_x number of people started with at birth and this quantity is known as the *Expectation of life at birth.*

Construction of a Life Table

In a life table, the q_x is the first column to be completed and this is obtained usually by the age and sex specific mortality rates at each age x. This column is called as the pivotal column of the life table.

An approximate value of q_x is obtained from the formula

$$q_x = \frac{2m_x}{2 + m_x}$$

Where m_x, is the age and sex specific death rates for the community at age x.

This formula has certain limitations as it assumes that the deaths are evenly distributed between any two successive ages. This is not true specifically in the early years of age when the deaths are more common in the first few weeks of birth than in the other weeks.

It is always better to take the estimated death rate by sample registration instead of the rates based on the routine registration data as it is known that the registration system in India is not very effective.

More elaborate formula are available for estimating q_x, at younger ages.

An extract from the All India Life Table for the decade 1961–70, for males is depicted in the Table 17.1 as an illustration. This is single year classification Life Table. Abridged Life Tables for five or ten year intervals are also prepared.

Life Table method is very useful in understanding survival rates from certain chronic diseases, as illustrated in the next Chapter.

Table 17.1: Life table of India for males during 1961-70

Age	No.living at age x	Mortality rate at age x	No.livng between ages x and x+1	Person years lived beyond the age x	Expectation of life at age x
X	l_x	q_x	L_x	T_x	e_x^0
0	100000	0.13500	89875	4707583	47.1
1	86500	0.04056	84430	4617708	53.4
2	82992	0.01256	82470	4533278	54.6
3	81950	0.00685	81668	4450808	54.3
4	81388	0.00578	81149	4369140	53.7
5	80918	0.00491	80720	4287991	53.0
6	80521	0.00423	80351	4207271	52.3
7	80181	0.00373	80032	4126920	51.5
8	79882	0.00341	79746	4046888	50.7
9	79609	0.00328	79479	3967142	49.8
10	79348	0.00302	79229	3887663	49.0
11	79109	0.00264	79004	3808434	48.1
12	78900	0.00245	78803	3729430	47.3
13	78706	0.00244	78611	3650627	46.4
14	78514	0.00260	78411	3572016	45.5
15	78309	0.00276	78201	3493605	44.6
16	78092	0.00278	77984	3415404	43.7
17	77875	0.00258	77764	3337420	42.9
18	77653	0.00297	77538	3259656	42.0
19	77422	0.00312	77301	3182118	41.1
20	77181	0.00314	77060	3104817	40.2
21	76938	0.00324	76813	3027757	39.4
22	76689	0.00333	76561	2950944	38.5
23	76433	0.00373	76065	2874383	37.6
24	76148	0.00434	75983	2798318	36.7
25	75818	0.00493	75632	2722335	35.9
26	75445	0.00538	75242	2646703	35.1
27	75039	0.00586	74820	2571461	34.3
28	74599	0.00636	74363	2496641	33.5
29	74125	0.00689	73871	2422278	32.7
30	73615	0.00693	73360	2348407	31.9
31	73105	0.00775	72822	2275047	31.1
32	72538	0.00851	72230	2202225	30.4
33	71921	0.00920	71591	2129995	29.6
34	71260	0.00983	70910	2058404	28.9
35	70559	0.01051	70189	1987494	28.2

contd...

contd...

Age	No.living at age x	Mortality rate at age x	No.livng between ages x and x+1	Person years lived beyond the age x	Expectation of life at age x
X	l_x	q_x	L_x	T_x	e_x^0
36	69818	0.01126	69425	1917305	27.5
37	69032	0.01188	68622	1847880	26.8
38	68212	0.01245	67787	1779258	26.1
39	67362	0.01295	66926	1711471	25.4
40	66490	0.01327	66049	1644545	24.7
41	65607	0.01365	65159	1578496	24.1
42	64711	0.01428	64249	1513337	23.4
43	63787	0.01515	63304	1449088	22.7
44	62821	0.01627	62310	1385784	22.1
45	61799	0.01724	61266	1323474	21.4
46	60733	0.01804	60185	1262208	20.8
47	59637	0.01907	59068	1202023	20.2
48	58500	0.02032	57905	1142955	19.5
49	57311	0.02180	56687	1085050	18.9
50	56062	0.02318	55413	1028363	18.3
51	54763	0.02440	54095	972950	17.8
52	53426	0.02578	52737	918855	17.2
53	52049	0.02730	51338	866118	16.6
54	50627	0.02897	49894	814780	16.1
55	49161	0.02999	48424	764886	15.6
56	47687	0.03092	46950	716462	15.0
57	46212	0.03280	45455	669512	14.5
58	44697	0.03563	43901	624057	14.0
59	43105	0.03941	42255	580156	13.5
60	41406	0.04316	40512	537901	13.0
61	39618	0.04626	38702	497389	12.6
62	37786	0.04938	36853	458687	12.1
63	35920	0.05252	34977	421834	11.7
64	34034	0.05568	33087	386857	11.4
65	32139	0.05921	31188	353770	11.0
66	30236	0.06272	29288	322582	10.7
67	28340	0.06563	27410	293294	10.3
68	26480	0.06795	25580	265884	10.0
69	24680	0.06970	23821	240304	9.7
70	22960	0.07121	22142	216483	9.4

contd...

contd...

Age	No.living at age x	Mortality rate at age x	No.livng between ages x and x+1	Person years lived beyond the age x	Expectation of life at age x
X	l_x	q_x	L_x	T_x	e_x^0
71	21325	0.07310	20546	194341	9.1
72	19766	0.07533	19022	173795	8.8
73	18277	0.07788	17566	154773	8.5
74	16854	0.08076	16174	137207	8.1
75	15494	0.08342	14848	121033	7.8
76	14201	0.08584	13593	106185	7.5
77	12983	0.08858	12408	92592	7.1
78	11832	0.09165	11290	80184	6.8
79	10747	0.09503	10237	68894	6.4
80	9726	0.09818	9249	58657	6.0
81	8771	0.10110	8328	49408	5.6
82	7884	0.10434	7473	41080	5.2
83	7062	0.10788	6682	33607	4.8
84	6300	0.11174	5948	26925	4.3
85+	5597			20977	3.7

18 Chapter — Survival Analysis

Need for Survival Analysis in Clinical Studies

Survival analysis in clinical studies is an important technique to assess the effectiveness of a given treatment as well as to understand the outcome in a group of subjects, with respect to a given disease, with passage of time. It provides information on the probability of survival for a newly diagnosed patient, following the onset of disease. It also provides information on prognosis according to patient characteristics like age, sex etc, as well as disease characteristics like site, histology etc. and also with respect to methods of treatment. Survival analysis techniques are not only useful in morbidity studies, but are useful in all follow up studies assessing failure rates etc.

Concepts in Survival Analysis

In survival studies, a group of individuals with some common morbidity experience is followed-up from a well defined starting point from which the survival is calculated. In the estimation of survival rates, the fundamental concepts such as starting date, common closing date of the study and vital status of all individuals at common closing date are to be defined before the initiation of study. These concepts are explained below.

i. *Starting Date*

It is the date of commencement of observation for a group of individuals in the study. This varies according to the purpose of the study. Commonly used starting dates include date of first symptom, date of diagnosis, date of hospital registration or admission, date of beginning of treatment etc.

ii. *Common Closing Date*

It refers to the date of termination of the study. This has to be fixed-up prior to the initiation of the study. Each individual has to be followed-up till the termination of the study.

iii. *Vital Status at Common Closing Date*

The vital status of each individual who participates in the study has to be assessed at closing date. In survival studies, when the period of observation ends, some patients would still be alive with or without the disease. Some of the patients would have died either due to disease of interest or due to causes other than that under study and some patients would be lost from the study due to other reasons. Any observation in the study that terminates due to the outcome of interest is called a 'failure' and only such observation has complete follow-up. All others would have incomplete follow-up and are considered as *'censored'* observations.

iv. *Length of Follow-up*

The length of follow-up is an important component in survival analysis which is defined as the length of time between the date of start and the date at which the observation ends. It is expressed in any arbitrary units of interval in terms of days, months or years, depending on the nature of the disease. The unit is selected based on the natural history of the disease under consideration. In diseases with long natural history the unit could be years. If the disease being studied has a very short natural course, the unit could be expressed in terms of months or days.

Methods for Estimation of Survival Rates

There are a number of techniques to estimate *Overall survival rates* such as Direct method, Actuarial or Life-table method, and the Kaplan-Meier product-limit method. When calculating the overall survival from any disease one may not take into account the cause of death, as it is possible that a few patients under follow up may die due to causes other than the disease of interest. But it may also be important to know the survival statistics due to the cause of disease under study, which is given by *Net survival rate.* Net survival rates from a disease can be calculated in terms of *Cause-specific survival Rate* and *Relative survival Rate.*

Methods adopted for estimating the Overall Survival rates are outlined below.

i. *Direct Method*

This method is a simple way of summarising patient survival. The survival probability at a given time is estimated by the ratio between the number of survivors at the end of a specified interval and the number of observations at the beginning of the study. In this method, all the censored observations are not included for calculation of survival rate. Only those who have completed the follow-up time of a specified interval are included, for which the rates are being calculated.

Table 18.1: Follow-up data on breast cancer patients put on two different therapies

Patient No.	Age	Therapy	Date of diagnosis	Date of last contact	Vital status	Cause of death	Duration of survival Years	Months
6	66	S	Jun-79	Aug-79	D	O	0	2
26	40	S+R	Apr-83	Jul-83	D	B	0	3
4	65	S+R	Feb-78	Jul-78	D	B	0	5
12	57	S+R	Oct-80	Jun-81	D	B	0	8
14	63	S+R	Jan-81	Jan-82	D	B	1	0
33	70	S+R	Sep-84	Sep-85	D	O	1	0
13	64	S+R	Dec-80	Feb-82	D	B	1	2
34	47	S+R	Sep-84	Dec-85	D	B	1	3
35	67	S+R	Oct-84	Apr-86	D	O	1	6
39	59	S	May-85	Dec-86	D	B	1	6
40	71	S	Jun-85	Mar-87	A	-	1	9
38	60	S+R	Apr-85	Jul-87	A	-	2	3
36	58	S	Jan-85	Aug-87	A	-	2	7
15	62	S	Jan-81	Oct-83	D	B	2	9
37	75	S+R	Jan-85	Oct-87	A	-	2	9
22	49	S+R	Mar-82	May-85	D	B	3	2
31	51	S	May-84	Jul-87	A	-	3	2

contd...

contd...

Patient No.	Age	Therapy	Date of diagnosis	Date of last contact	Vital status	Cause of death	Duration of survival Years	Months
32	40	S	Jul-84	Nov-87	A	-	3	4
30	63	S+R	Apr-84	Nov-87	D	O	3	7
28	47	S+R	Jun-83	Feb-87	A	-	3	8
29	55	S	Jan-84	Nov-87	A	-	3	10
27	65	S+R	Apr-83	Oct-87	A	-	4	6
17	76	S	Jul-81	Feb-86	D	B	4	7
24	48	S	Oct-82	Jun-87	D	B	4	8
23	50	S	Jul-82	Apr-87	A	-	4	9
25	82	S	Mar-83	Dec-87	A	-	4	9
3	58	S+R	Sep-77	Aug-82	D	B	4	11
19	67	S+R	Nov-81	Feb-87	D	O	5	3
20	59	S	Nov-81	Apr-87	A	-	5	5
16	73	S	Apr-81	Feb-87	A	-	5	10
21	76	S	Dec-81	Sep-87	A	-	5	10
18	51	S+R	Sep-81	Nov-87	A	-	6	2
10	44	S	Apr-80	Jul-87	A	-	7	3
9	45	S+R	Mar-80	Jun-87	A	-	7	7
11	56	S+R	Apr-80	Oct-87	A	-	7	7
5	71	S	Feb-78	Nov-85	D	O	7	9
8	51	S	Oct-79	Nov-87	A	-	8	1
7	45	S+R	Jul-79	Dec-87	A	-	8	8
2	57	S	Apr-77	Apr-87	A	-	10	0
1	53	S	Jan-77	Nov-87	A	-	10	10

Note: Therapy : S: Only Surgery, S+ R : Surgery and Radio Therapy
Vital status : A : Alive, D : Dead
Cause of death : B : Breast Cancer, O : Other Causes

Example 18.1. Calculation of Observed Survival rate from Direct Method for the above data, for first three years is given below.

Patients numbered 6, 26, 4, and 12 died during the first year of follow up. So 36 patients survived beyond one year out of 40 followed up.

a. Survival rate for first year = (36 / 40) = 0.90 or 90%
b. Patients numbered 6, 26, 4, 12, 14, 33, 13, 34, 35 and 40 died during first and second year of follow up. So the remaining 30 patients survived beyond 2 years out of 40 followed-up. Survival rate for two years = (30 / 40) = 0.75 or 75%

c. Patients numbered 6, 26, 4, 12, 14, 33, 13, 34, 35, 39, 15, 22, and 30 died during first three years of follow up. So 27 survived beyond three years out of 40 followed up.

Survival rate for three years = (27 / 40) = 0.68 or 68%.

It can be seen that this method takes into account all the patients who were included in the study at the start for calculation of Survival rates at different periods and does not take into account all the censored observations and only those who completed the specified follow up time.

Standard Error (SE) of Survival rate calculated by Direct method is

$$SE(P) = \sqrt{[P(1-P)/N]}$$

Where, P is the Survival Rate

N is the number of subjects

Thus the Standard Error of Survival Rate at three years

$$= \sqrt{[(0.68)(0.32)/40]} = 0.07$$

ii. *Actuarial or Life-table Method*

In this method of calculating the survival, two types of censored observations, namely, patients who are lost to follow-up during observation period and those known to be alive but withdrawn from observations due to closure of the study are considered for calculation and necessary corrections are made for obtaining the number alive at the start of any interval. This method is frequently referred to as the 'Actuarial' method because the techniques used are similar to those employed by Actuaries. This method assumes that censored observations are subject to the same mortality conditions as those of patients with complete follow-up.

First step in the computation of survival rates by this method is the subdivision of the maximum follow-up survival time into some intervals of period set *in advance* based on the distribution of deaths over a period of time and the intervals may be of equal or unequal duration.

The second step is the calculation of number of observations exposed to the risk of dying (N_i), known as effective number at risk at any interval and is calculated as:

$$N_i = [n_i - (w_i / 2)]$$

where,

w_i is the no.of patients last seen alive during interval including withdrawals.

n_i is the number of patients at the start of the interval.

The third step is the computation of probabilities of death (q_i) in each interval , calculated as :

$$(q_i = d_i / N_i).$$

where,

N_i is the effective number of patients at risk as calculated above.

d_i is the number of patients dying during the interval.

Then the probability of survival (p_i) during each interval is calculated as $p_i = (1 - q_i)$.

The survival rate at the end of a given interval 'i' is obtained by multiplying the probabilities of survival over all the intervals preceding and up to this time interval and is obtained as

$(P_i = p_1 \times p_2 \times \ldots\ldots\ldots \times p_i)$ and is called *Cumulative survival rate.*

Example 18.2. Calculation of observed survival rate by this method for the data given in Table 18.1 is demonstrated in Table 18.2.

Table 18.2: Tabular presentation for calculation of observed survival rate by Actuarial method

Interval in months after diagnosis	No. of patients alive at beginning of interval	No. of patients dying during the interval	No. Last seen alive during interval (With-drawal)	Effective No. exposed to risk of dying	Proport-tion dying during interval	Proport- surviving the interval	Cumulative proportion surviving (Survival rate at the end of interval)
I	N_i	d_i	w_i	$n_i = (N_i - \frac{W_i}{2})$	$q_i = (d_i/n_i)$	$p_i = (1 - q_i)$	P_i
0	40	4	0	40.0	0.100	0.900	0.9000
12	36	6	1	35.5	0.169	0.831	0.7479
24	29	1	3	27.5	0.036	0.964	0.7207
36	25	2	4	23.0	0.087	0.913	0.6580
48	19	3	3	17.5	0.171	0.829	0.5452
60	13	1	3	11.5	0.087	0.913	0.4978
72 +	9	0	1	8.5	0.000	1.000	0.4978

Survival rate at the end of 48 months is 0.5452 or 54.52%, while at 72+ months is 0.4978 or 49.78 %.

Standard Error of the Cumulative Survival Rate is obtained from the formula

$$SE(P_i) = (P_i)\sqrt{[\Sigma\{q_i/(n_i - d_i)\}]}$$

Where, P_i = Survival rate at interval i

n_i = Effective No. exposed to the risk at the start of interval i

d_i = No. of events during interval i

q_i = Proportion of events happening during the interval I

The calculation of Standard Error of estimates of P_i for different intervals is demonstrated in a Tabular form under Table 18.3.

Example 18.3.

Table 18.3: Calculation of standard error for estimates of survival rate obtained by actuarial method.

Effective no. exposed to the risk n_i	No. dying during the interval d_i	$(n_i - d_i)$	Proportion dying during the interval q_i	$q_i/(n_i-d_i)$	Cum total of (q_i/n_i-d_i)	Square root of Cum. Tot. of (q_i/n_i-d_i)	Survival rate at the end of interval	Standard error of survival rate
40	4	36.0	0.100	0.0028	0.0028	0.053	0.9000	0.0477
35.5	6	29.5	0.169	0.0057	0.0085	0.092	0.7479	0.0688
27.5	1	26.5	0.036	0.0014	0.0099	0.099	0.7207	0.0713
23	2	21.0	0.087	0.0041	0.0140	0.118	0.6580	0.0776
17.5	3	14.5	0.171	0.0118	0.0259	0.161	0.5452	0.0878
11.5	1	10.5	0.087	0.0083	0.0342	0.185	0.4978	0.0921
8.5	0	8.5	0.000	0.0000	0.0342	0.185	0.4978	0.0921
6.5	1	5.5	0.154	0.0280	0.0621	0.249	0.4212	0.1049
3	0	3.0	0.000	0.0000	0.0621	0.249	0.4212	0.1049

iii. *Kaplan-Meier or Product-Limit Method*

This is a modified method to Actuarial method described above. Here the time intervals of observation are determined by the occurrence of outcome of event, commonly as months, as and when they occur in contrast to the Actuarial method in which there was a need for grouping the data in pre-fixed time intervals. The follow-up time of all observations in the study are arranged in increasing order of magnitude. The procedure followed is the same as that of Actuarial method except that patients withdrawn from observation are considered to have survived throughout the time period in which they occur.

Number of patients alive at the beginning of any month, n_i is obtained as the difference between the number alive at the beginning of previous month and the total of deaths and withdrawals in the previous month as calculated below.

n_i for second month = n_i for first month - (No. of death and withdrawals in first month)

The conditional probabilities of survival at ith interval is estimated every time an event occurs in that interval. As in the Actuarial method, the cumulative survival rate (cp_i)at any given time point is obtained by the product of all conditional probabilities of survival calculated at each event up to the time point under consideration.

cp_i of survival at ith interval =

(cp_i of the previous interval) (p_i of the ith interval)

This method requires the calculation of as many survival rates as there are events, except if several events occur on the same time. Hence this method is also called as *Product-limit method.*

If there are no events, rates are not calculated for that month. Thus survival rate at the end of 15 months is 0.80 or 80%, while at the end of 63 months is 0.5042 or 50.42%.

Survival curve consisting of horizontal lines with vertical steps corresponding to each event, can be plotted and is known as *Step-ladder*. The horizontal lines correspond to each event and the vertical axis of the graph represents the survival rate for members of the study group. The magnitude of the step is related to the number of observations at risk and the number of events occurring. The points on the survival curve are the best estimate of the survival rates for members of the study group.

The survival rates at the beginning of the curve are more definite and reliable in both the Actuarial and the Kaplan-Meier method, because a higher number of observations are at risk

Table 18.4: Calculation of observed survival rate for data on 40 female patients with breast cancer given in Table 18.1, by the Kaplan-Meier method

Month after diagnosis i	Number alive at beginning of the month N_1	No. of deaths in the month d_i	No. of withdrawal in the month w_1	Proportion dying in the month $q_i = (d_i/n_i)$	Proportion surviving the month $p_i = (1 - qi)$	Cumulative surviving from treatment cpi= $cp_{(i-1)} P_i$
2	40	1	0	0.025	0.975	
3	39	1	0	0.026	0.974	0.9750
5	38	1	0	0.026	0.974	0.9500
8	37	1	0	0.027	0.973	0.9250
12	36	2	0	0.056	0.944	0.9000
14	34	1	0	0.029	0.971	0.8500
15	33	1	0	0.030	0.970	0.8250
18	32	2	0	0.063	0.938	0.8000
21	30	0	1			0.7500
27	29	0	1			0.7500
31	28	0	1			0.7500
33	27	1	1	0.037	0.963	0.7500
38	25	1	1	0.040	0.960	
40	23	0	1			0.7222
43	22	1	0	0.045	0.955	
44	21	0	1			0.6618
46	20	0	1			
54	19	0	1			
55	18	1	0	0.056	0.944	
56	17	1	0	0.059	0.941	0.6251
57	16	0	2			0.5883
59	14	1	0	0.071	0.929	
63	13	1	0	0.077	0.923	0.5463
65	12	0	1			0.5042
69	11	0	1			
70	10	0	1			
74	9	0	1			
87	8	0	2			
90	6	0	1			
93	5	1	0	0.200	0.800	
97	4	0	1			0.4034
101	3	0	1			
120	2	0	1			
130	1	0	1			

during these time intervals. However, at the tail end of the curve, the number of observations at risk is relatively small because of increased censored observations resulting in fewer patients being followed-up for that length of time.

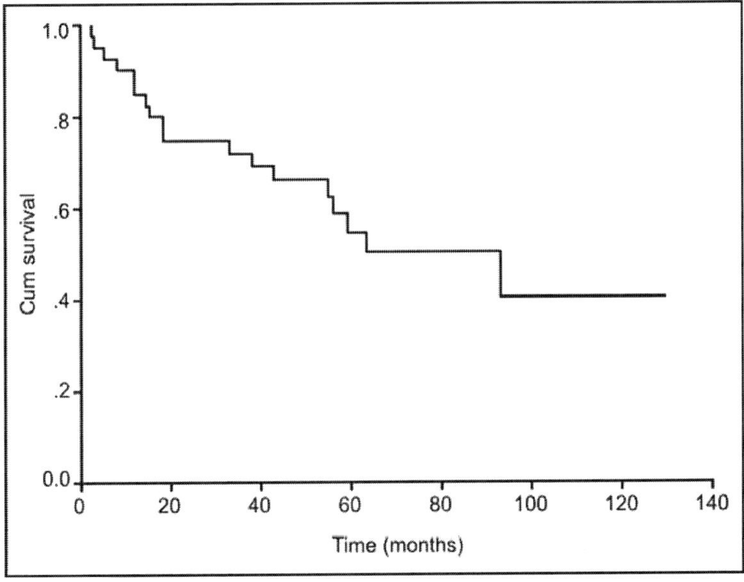

Fig. 18.1: Overall survival curve by Kaplan-Meier method

A rough estimate of the Standard error of Survival rate P_i estimated by Kaplan-Meier method at the end of a given interval (i) is obtained as :

$$SE(p_i) = (p_i)\sqrt{[(1 - p_i) / n_i]}$$

Where

n_i is the number of cases at risk at interval i

p_i is the survival rate at interval i.

On the assumption that p_i will follow approximately Normal distribution, 95% confidence interval would be $p_i \pm 1.96$ SE (p_i)

Example 18.5. In the previous Example, the survival rate at, say, 15 months was 0.800 with 33 patients at risk at that interval.

Standard Error of Survival rate at 15 months

$$= (0.800)\sqrt{[(1 - 0.800) / 33]}$$

$$= (0.800)\ \sqrt{(0.200/33)}$$
$$= (0.800)\ (0.078) = 0.062$$

The confidence interval for the survival rate at 18 months is

$$= 0.800 \pm 1.96\ (0.062) = 0.800 \pm 0.122$$

Thus the confidence interval for survival rate at 15 months would be

0.922 to 0.678.

a. *Mean Survival Time*

Mean survival time is the average duration of the follow-up time of all observations in the study. To estimate mean survival time accurately, all individuals must have 'complete follow-up time'. i.e. all observations must be 'failures' by the closure of the study. Otherwise, the estimate of mean survival time is based on incomplete observations (censored) and does not reflect a true picture of the data.

b. *Median Survival Time*

It is the time at which the survival rate is equal to fifty percent. This can be estimated from the survival curve plotted by using either the Actuarial or the Kaplan-Meier method.

Methods for Estimation of Net Survival

All deaths occurring among subjects being followed up, including deaths from causes other than the disease of interest, are considered as 'failures' in the calculation of overall survival rate using the above methods. Thus the probability of survival computed by above methods is a sum of two components, one due to deaths attributable to the disease under study and the other due to deaths because of other causes. As such it is essential to understand the 'Net survival' attributable to only the disease under study. The Net survival probabilities are useful to make comparisons between subpopulations from the same region or between populations from different regions where the mortality due to other causes may be different. To describe the deaths attributable only to the disease under study, the method of cause-specific survival or the method of relative survival can be used as described below.

i. *Cause-specific Survival*

When reliable information on the causes of death of all subjects are available, Cause-specific survival can be obtained by considering only those cases for which cause of death other than the disease under study is considered as 'censored' observations. i.e. only those deaths occurring due to the disease of interest are considered as failures while other deaths are considered as simply termination of follow-up, in the same way as cases lost to follow-up or withdrawn alive. The estimation of cause-specific survival can be carried out by the Actuarial method or by the Kaplan-Meier method, after making this correction.

ii. *Relative Survival*

The method of relative survival does not require knowledge on the cause of death and thus avoids the difficulties associated with the determination of cause of death. Relative survival is calculated as a ratio of the *overall survival as per the study* to the *expected survival* in the general population, if it had the same distribution pattern, of a factor to be controlled, as that of the study population. As an example, if age is considered as a factor to be controlled, the expected survival is obtained as the number of survivors, which can be predicted at time 't' in a population having the same age structure as that of the disease group under study, but subject to the conditions of mortality in the general population. Expected number of survivors is calculated first for each subgroup defined by the age at diagnosis in single years or by larger age groups using the available life tables. Number of deaths calculated as above, for each age interval is summed up to get the expected number of deaths under the mortality conditions as it exists in the general population. This method of calculation is similar to the one described under standardisation of rates.

The method of relative survival is based on the assumption that the general mortality, as is described by the Life-table of the population, adequately takes into account of all causes of mortality, except for the specific cause under study. The cause due to disease of interest is considered negligible in comparison to all other causes of death. Only on this condition, Relative survival can provide an acceptable approximation to Net survival. If this assumption does not hold, Net survival will be overestimated as a result of the increased estimation of the mortality due to other causes.

Life-tables published by Census Organisation or Sample Registration System of Government of India are usually available to calculate expected survival in our country. However, when Life table suitable for the population being studied is not available, due the fact that the population being followed is too selected for the mortality to be described by the official table, a table can be constructed from available mortality rates, provided these rates are sufficiently reliable and accurate.

Methods for Comparing the Survival Rates

Survival rates between any two groups can be compared at any time point on the survival curve. Further, tests like Rank tests or Stratified analysis tests can be used for comparing the survival experience of different levels of one prognostic factor with the other. Cox-regression model, can also be used to compare a number of prognostic factors, especially when stratified analysis cannot be applied due to the fact that strata sizes are small.

i. *Z-Test to Compare Two Survival Rates*

The standard Z-test provides an estimate of the probability that a difference between two survival rates as large as that observed would have occurred only due to sampling variation. .

If p_1 and p_2 are the survival rates at any point of time, for two groups 1 and 2, and SE (p_1) and SE (p_2) are the standard errors for p_1 and p_2 respectively then the statistic Z, is calculated by the following formula, as already illustrated under Chapter 12.

$$Z = | (p_1 - p_2) | \ / \ \sqrt{[SE^2 (p_1) + SE^2 (p_2)]}$$

where, $|(p_1 - p_2)|$ is the absolute value of the difference of survival rates.

If the observed value of Z for a particular set of data is equal to or more than 1.96, then it can be concluded that a difference, as large as that observed, is due to sampling variation, with a probability of five percent or less.

ii. *Log- Rank Test to Compare Survival Curves*

The difference between two or more survival curves can be tested by Rank tests. Commonly used rank test is *Log-rank test*. This test is designed particularly to detect a difference between two or more survival rates when the mortality rate in one group is consistently higher than the corresponding rate in another group and the ratio of these two rates is constant over time.

If O_1 and O_2 are the observed number of deaths in two groups 1 and 2 and E_1 and E_2 are the corresponding expected number of deaths, then the log-rank statistic (T) used for comparison purposes is obtained as :

$$T = [(O_1 - E_1)^2 / E_1 + (O_2 - E_2)^2 / E_2]$$

Based on the number of individuals in each group who are alive just before any point of interval and the total number of deaths observed at that point of interval in both the groups, expected number of deaths in each group can be calculated, under null hypothesis. Total number of deaths in both the groups is proportioned according to the number of patients observed in each group. If the null hypothesis is true, T is approximately distributed as a Chi-square distribution with one degree of freedom. i.e. if the calculated value of T for a particular set of data is equal to or more than 3.84, then the probability that a difference as that observed between the two groups is due to sampling variation is 5% or less.

iii. *Stratified Comparison of Survival*

The survival of a group of patients is generally associated with many prognostic factors which are inter-related. The comparison should take these prognostic factors into account by a method based on an appropriate stratification, provided that the necessary information is available for each subject. Employing stratified rank test, the survival experience of different levels of one factor, can be assessed after adjusting for other prognostic factors. Computer programmes for these tests are available in all major Statistical Software packages which makes the application of these procedures easier.

iv. *Regression Models*

Cox in 1972 developed a modelling procedure called the Cox-proportional hazards model for use when the number of prognostic factors is large. The model helps to assess the effect of various prognostic factors on survival after adjusting for factors with each other. In other words, through this approach, it is possible to identify the independent prognostic factors associated with the survival. The advantage of the procedure is that it does not assume a specific mathematical distribution for observed failures over time. The model measures hazard ratio of outcome under the assumption that the hazard is constant over the follow-up period.

Statistical Software packages are available for application of these models.

Appendix 1: Table of normal probability integrals

Z		0	1	2	3	4	5	6	7	8	9
0.0	0.	5000	49601	49202	48803	48405	48006	47608	47210	46812	46414
0.1		46017	45620	45224	44828	44433	44038	43644	43251	42858	43465
0.2		42074	41683	41294	40905	40517	40129	39743	39358	38974	38591
0.3		38209	37828	37448	37070	36693	36317	35942	35569	35197	34827
0.4		34458	34090	33724	33360	32997	32636	32276	31918	31561	31207
0.5		30854	30503	30153	29806	29460	29116	28774	28434	28096	27760
0.6		27425	27093	26763	26435	26109	25785	25463	25143	24825	24510
0.7		24196	23885	23576	23270	22965	22663	22363	22065	21770	21476
0.8		21186	20897	20611	20327	20045	19766	19489	19215	18943	18673
0.9		18406	18141	17879	17619	17361	17106	16853	16602	16354	16109
1.0		15866	15625	15386	15151	14917	14686	14457	14231	14007	13786
1.1		13567	13350	13136	12924	12714	12507	12302	12100	11900	11702
1.2		11507	11314	11123	10935	10749	10 565	10383	10204	10027	98525
1.3	0.0	96800	95098	93418	91759	90123	88508	86915	85343	83793	82264
1.4		80757	79270	77804	76359	74934	73529	72145	70781	69437	68112
1.5		66807	65522	64255	63008	61780	60571	59380	58208	57053	55917
1.6		54799	53699	52616	51551	50503	49471	48457	47460	46479	45514
1.7		44565	43633	42716	41815	40930	40059	39204	38364	37538	36727
1.8		35930	35148	34380	33625	32884	32157	31443	30742	30054	29379
1.9		28717	28067	27429	26803	26190	25588	24998	24419	23852	23295
2.0		22750	22216	21692	21178	20675	20182	19699	19226	18763	18309
2.1		17864	17429	17003	16586	16177	15778	15386	15003	14629	14262
2.2		13903	13553	13209	12874	12545	12224	11911	11604	11304	11011
2.3		10724	10444	10170	99031	96419	93867	91375	88940	86563	84242

contd...

Z	0	1	2	3	4	5	6	7	8	9
2.4	0.0^2 81975	79763	77603	75494	73436	71428	69469	67557	65691	63872
2.5	62097	60366	58677	57031	55426	53861	52336	50849	49400	47988
2.6	46612	45271	43965	42692	41453	40246	39070	37926	36811	35726
2.7	34670	33642	32641	31667	30720	29798	28901	28028	27179	26354
2.8	25551	24771	24012	23274	22557	21860	21182	20524	19884	19262
2.9	18658	18071	17502	16948	16411	15889	15382	14890	14412	13949
3.0	13499	13062	12639	12228	11829	11442	11067	10703	10350	10008
3.1	0.0^3 96760	93544	90426	87403	84474	81635	78885	76219	73638	71136
3.2	68714	66367	64095	61895	59765	57703	55706	53774	51904	50094
3.3	48342	46648	45009	43423	41889	40406	38971	37584	36243	34946
3.4	33693	32481	31311	30179	29086	28029	27009	26023	25071	24151
3.5	23263	22405	21577	20778	20006	19262	18543	17849	17180	16534
3.6	15911	15310	14730	14171	13632	13112	12611	12128	11662	11213
3.7	10780	10363	99611	95740	92010	88417	84957	81624	78414	75324
3.8	0.0^4 72348	69483	66726	64072	61517	59059	56694	54418	52228	50122
3.9	48096	46148	44274	42473	40741	39076	37475	35936	34458	33037
4.0	31671	30359	29099	27888	26726	25609	24536	23507	22518	21569
4.1	20658	19783	18944	18138	17365	16624	15912	15230	14575	13948
4.2	13346	12769	12215	11685	11176	10689	10221	97736	93447	89337
4.3	0.0^5 85399	81627	78015	74555	71241	68069	65031	62123	59340	56675
4.4	54125	51685	49350	47117	44979	42935	40980	39110	37322	35612
4.5	33977	32414	30920	29492	28127	26823	25577	24386	23249	22162
4.6	21125	20133	19187	18283	17420	16597	15810	15060	14344	13660
4.7	13008	12386	11792	11226	10686	10171	96796	92113	87648	83391
4.8	0.0^6 79333	75465	71779	68267	64920	61731	58693	55799	53043	50418
4.9	47918	45538	43272	41115	39061	37107	35247	33476	31792	30190

Appendix 2: Table of random numbers

<table>
<tr><td>53</td><td>74</td><td>23</td><td>99</td><td>67</td><td>61</td><td>32</td><td>28</td><td>69</td><td>84</td><td>94</td><td>62</td><td>67</td><td>86</td><td>24</td><td>98</td><td>33</td><td>41</td><td>19</td><td>95</td><td>47</td><td>53</td><td>53</td><td>38</td><td>09</td></tr>
<tr><td>63</td><td>38</td><td>06</td><td>86</td><td>54</td><td>99</td><td>00</td><td>65</td><td>26</td><td>94</td><td>02</td><td>82</td><td>90</td><td>23</td><td>07</td><td>79</td><td>62</td><td>67</td><td>80</td><td>60</td><td>75</td><td>91</td><td>12</td><td>81</td><td>19</td></tr>
<tr><td>35</td><td>30</td><td>58</td><td>21</td><td>46</td><td>06</td><td>72</td><td>17</td><td>10</td><td>94</td><td>25</td><td>21</td><td>31</td><td>75</td><td>96</td><td>49</td><td>28</td><td>24</td><td>00</td><td>49</td><td>55</td><td>65</td><td>79</td><td>78</td><td>07</td></tr>
<tr><td>63</td><td>43</td><td>36</td><td>82</td><td>69</td><td>65</td><td>51</td><td>18</td><td>37</td><td>88</td><td>61</td><td>38</td><td>44</td><td>12</td><td>45</td><td>32</td><td>92</td><td>85</td><td>88</td><td>65</td><td>54</td><td>34</td><td>81</td><td>85</td><td>35</td></tr>
<tr><td>98</td><td>25</td><td>37</td><td>55</td><td>26</td><td>01</td><td>91</td><td>82</td><td>81</td><td>46</td><td>74</td><td>71</td><td>12</td><td>94</td><td>97</td><td>24</td><td>02</td><td>71</td><td>37</td><td>07</td><td>03</td><td>92</td><td>18</td><td>66</td><td>75</td></tr>
<tr><td>02</td><td>63</td><td>21</td><td>17</td><td>69</td><td>71</td><td>50</td><td>80</td><td>89</td><td>56</td><td>38</td><td>15</td><td>70</td><td>11</td><td>48</td><td>43</td><td>40</td><td>45</td><td>86</td><td>98</td><td>00</td><td>83</td><td>26</td><td>91</td><td>03</td></tr>
<tr><td>64</td><td>55</td><td>22</td><td>21</td><td>82</td><td>48</td><td>22</td><td>28</td><td>06</td><td>00</td><td>61</td><td>54</td><td>13</td><td>43</td><td>91</td><td>82</td><td>78</td><td>12</td><td>23</td><td>29</td><td>06</td><td>66</td><td>24</td><td>12</td><td>27</td></tr>
<tr><td>85</td><td>07</td><td>26</td><td>13</td><td>89</td><td>01</td><td>10</td><td>07</td><td>82</td><td>04</td><td>59</td><td>63</td><td>69</td><td>36</td><td>03</td><td>69</td><td>11</td><td>15</td><td>83</td><td>80</td><td>13</td><td>29</td><td>54</td><td>19</td><td>28</td></tr>
<tr><td>58</td><td>54</td><td>16</td><td>24</td><td>15</td><td>51</td><td>54</td><td>44</td><td>82</td><td>00</td><td>62</td><td>61</td><td>65</td><td>04</td><td>69</td><td>38</td><td>18</td><td>65</td><td>18</td><td>97</td><td>85</td><td>72</td><td>13</td><td>49</td><td>21</td></tr>
<tr><td>34</td><td>85</td><td>27</td><td>84</td><td>87</td><td>61</td><td>48</td><td>64</td><td>56</td><td>26</td><td>90</td><td>18</td><td>48</td><td>13</td><td>26</td><td>37</td><td>70</td><td>15</td><td>42</td><td>57</td><td>65</td><td>65</td><td>80</td><td>39</td><td>07</td></tr>
<tr><td>03</td><td>92</td><td>18</td><td>27</td><td>46</td><td>57</td><td>99</td><td>16</td><td>96</td><td>56</td><td>30</td><td>33</td><td>72</td><td>85</td><td>22</td><td>84</td><td>64</td><td>38</td><td>56</td><td>98</td><td>99</td><td>01</td><td>30</td><td>98</td><td>64</td></tr>
<tr><td>62</td><td>95</td><td>30</td><td>27</td><td>59</td><td>37</td><td>75</td><td>41</td><td>66</td><td>48</td><td>86</td><td>97</td><td>80</td><td>61</td><td>45</td><td>23</td><td>53</td><td>04</td><td>01</td><td>63</td><td>45</td><td>76</td><td>08</td><td>64</td><td>27</td></tr>
<tr><td>08</td><td>45</td><td>93</td><td>15</td><td>22</td><td>60</td><td>21</td><td>75</td><td>46</td><td>91</td><td>98</td><td>77</td><td>27</td><td>85</td><td>42</td><td>28</td><td>88</td><td>61</td><td>08</td><td>84</td><td>69</td><td>62</td><td>03</td><td>42</td><td>73</td></tr>
<tr><td>07</td><td>08</td><td>55</td><td>18</td><td>40</td><td>45</td><td>44</td><td>75</td><td>13</td><td>90</td><td>24</td><td>94</td><td>96</td><td>61</td><td>02</td><td>57</td><td>55</td><td>66</td><td>83</td><td>15</td><td>73</td><td>42</td><td>37</td><td>11</td><td>61</td></tr>
<tr><td>01</td><td>85</td><td>89</td><td>95</td><td>66</td><td>51</td><td>10</td><td>19</td><td>34</td><td>88</td><td>15</td><td>84</td><td>97</td><td>19</td><td>75</td><td>12</td><td>76</td><td>39</td><td>43</td><td>78</td><td>64</td><td>63</td><td>91</td><td>08</td><td>25</td></tr>
<tr><td>72</td><td>84</td><td>71</td><td>14</td><td>35</td><td>19</td><td>11</td><td>58</td><td>49</td><td>26</td><td>50</td><td>11</td><td>17</td><td>17</td><td>76</td><td>86</td><td>31</td><td>57</td><td>20</td><td>18</td><td>95</td><td>60</td><td>78</td><td>46</td><td>75</td></tr>
<tr><td>88</td><td>78</td><td>28</td><td>16</td><td>84</td><td>13</td><td>52</td><td>53</td><td>94</td><td>53</td><td>75</td><td>45</td><td>69</td><td>30</td><td>96</td><td>73</td><td>89</td><td>65</td><td>70</td><td>31</td><td>99</td><td>17</td><td>43</td><td>48</td><td>76</td></tr>
<tr><td>45</td><td>17</td><td>75</td><td>65</td><td>57</td><td>28</td><td>40</td><td>19</td><td>72</td><td>12</td><td>25</td><td>12</td><td>74</td><td>75</td><td>67</td><td>60</td><td>40</td><td>60</td><td>81</td><td>19</td><td>24</td><td>62</td><td>01</td><td>61</td><td>16</td></tr>
<tr><td>96</td><td>76</td><td>28</td><td>12</td><td>54</td><td>22</td><td>01</td><td>11</td><td>95</td><td>25</td><td>71</td><td>96</td><td>16</td><td>16</td><td>88</td><td>68</td><td>64</td><td>36</td><td>74</td><td>45</td><td>19</td><td>59</td><td>50</td><td>88</td><td>92</td></tr>
<tr><td>43</td><td>31</td><td>67</td><td>72</td><td>30</td><td>24</td><td>02</td><td>94</td><td>08</td><td>63</td><td>38</td><td>32</td><td>36</td><td>66</td><td>02</td><td>69</td><td>36</td><td>38</td><td>25</td><td>39</td><td>48</td><td>03</td><td>45</td><td>15</td><td>22</td></tr>
<tr><td>50</td><td>44</td><td>66</td><td>44</td><td>21</td><td>66</td><td>06</td><td>58</td><td>05</td><td>62</td><td>68</td><td>15</td><td>54</td><td>35</td><td>02</td><td>42</td><td>35</td><td>48</td><td>96</td><td>32</td><td>14</td><td>52</td><td>41</td><td>52</td><td>48</td></tr>
<tr><td>22</td><td>66</td><td>22</td><td>15</td><td>86</td><td>26</td><td>63</td><td>75</td><td>41</td><td>99</td><td>58</td><td>42</td><td>36</td><td>72</td><td>24</td><td>58</td><td>37</td><td>52</td><td>18</td><td>51</td><td>03</td><td>37</td><td>18</td><td>39</td><td>11</td></tr>
<tr><td>96</td><td>24</td><td>40</td><td>14</td><td>51</td><td>23</td><td>22</td><td>30</td><td>88</td><td>57</td><td>95</td><td>67</td><td>47</td><td>29</td><td>83</td><td>94</td><td>69</td><td>40</td><td>06</td><td>07</td><td>18</td><td>16</td><td>36</td><td>78</td><td>86</td></tr>
<tr><td>31</td><td>73</td><td>91</td><td>61</td><td>19</td><td>60</td><td>20</td><td>72</td><td>93</td><td>48</td><td>98</td><td>57</td><td>07</td><td>23</td><td>69</td><td>65</td><td>95</td><td>39</td><td>69</td><td>58</td><td>56</td><td>80</td><td>30</td><td>19</td><td>44</td></tr>
<tr><td>78</td><td>60</td><td>73</td><td>99</td><td>84</td><td>43</td><td>89</td><td>94</td><td>36</td><td>45</td><td>56</td><td>69</td><td>94</td><td>36</td><td>45</td><td>90</td><td>22</td><td>91</td><td>07</td><td>12</td><td>78</td><td>35</td><td>34</td><td>08</td><td>72</td></tr>
</table>

contd...

84	37	90	61	56	70	10	23	98	05	85	11	34	76	60	76	48	45	34	60	01	64	18	39	96
36	67	10	08	23	98	93	35	08	86	99	29	76	29	81	33	34	91	58	93	63	14	52	32	52
07	28	59	07	48	89	64	58	89	75	83	85	62	27	89	30	14	78	56	27	86	63	59	80	02
10	15	83	87	60	79	24	31	66	56	21	48	24	06	93	91	98	94	05	49	01	47	59	38	00
55	19	68	97	65	03	73	52	16	56	00	53	55	90	27	33	42	29	38	87	22	13	88	83	34
53	81	29	13	39	35	01	20	71	34	62	33	74	82	14	53	73	19	09	03	56	54	29	56	93
51	86	32	68	92	33	98	74	66	99	40	14	71	94	58	45	94	19	38	81	14	44	99	81	07
35	91	70	29	13	80	03	54	07	27	96	94	78	32	66	50	95	52	74	33	13	80	55	62	54
37	71	67	95	13	20	02	44	95	94	64	85	04	05	72	01	32	90	76	14	53	89	74	60	41
93	66	13	83	27	92	79	64	64	72	28	54	96	53	84	48	14	52	98	94	56	07	93	89	30
02	96	08	45	65	13	05	00	41	84	93	07	54	72	59	21	45	57	09	77	19	48	56	27	44
49	83	43	48	35	82	88	33	69	96	72	36	04	19	76	47	45	15	18	60	82	11	08	95	97
84	60	71	62	46	40	80	81	30	37	34	39	23	05	38	25	15	35	71	30	88	12	57	21	77
18	17	30	88	71	44	91	14	88	47	89	23	30	63	15	56	34	20	47	89	99	82	93	24	98
79	69	10	61	78	71	32	76	95	62	87	00	22	58	40	92	54	01	75	25	43	11	71	99	31
75	93	36	57	83	56	20	14	82	11	74	21	97	90	65	96	42	68	63	86	74	54	13	26	94
38	30	92	29	03	06	28	81	39	38	62	25	06	84	63	61	29	08	93	67	04	32	92	08	00
51	29	50	10	34	31	57	75	95	80	51	97	02	74	77	76	15	48	49	44	18	55	63	77	09
21	31	38	86	24	37	79	81	53	74	73	24	16	10	33	52	83	90	94	76	70	47	14	54	36
29	01	23	87	88	58	02	39	37	67	42	10	14	20	92	16	55	23	42	45	54	96	09	11	06
95	33	95	22	00	18	74	72	00	18	38	79	58	69	32	81	76	80	26	92	82	80	84	25	39
90	84	60	79	80	24	36	59	87	38	82	07	53	89	35	96	35	23	79	18	05	98	90	07	35

Appendix 3: Table of t-distribution

n	0.90	0.80	0.70	0.60	0.50	0.40	0.30	0.20	0.10	0.05	0.02	0.01	0.001
1	0.158	0.325	0.510	0.727	1.000	1.376	1.963	3.078	6.314	12.706	31.821	63.657	636.619
2	0.142	0.289	0.445	0.617	0.816	1.061	1.386	1.886	2.920	4.303	6.965	9.925	31.598
3	0.137	0.277	0.424	0.584	0.765	0.978	1.250	1.638	2.353	3.182	4.541	5.841	12.924
4	0.134	0.271	0.414	0.569	0.741	0.941	1.190	1.533	2.132	2.776	3.747	4.604	8.61
5	0.132	0.267	0.408	0.559	0.727	0.920	1.156	1.476	2.015	2.571	3.365	4.032	6.869
6	0.131	0.265	0.404	0.553	0.718	0.906	1.134	1.440	1.943	2.447	3.143	3.707	5.959
7	0.130	0.263	0.402	0.549	0.711	0.896	1.119	1.415	1.895	2.365	2.998	3.499	5.408
8	0.130	0.262	0.399	0.546	0.706	0.889	1.108	1.397	1.860	2.306	2.896	3.355	5.041
9	0.129	0.260	0.398	0.543	0.703	0.883	1.100	1.383	1.833	2.262	2.821	3.250	4.781
10	0.129	0.260	0.397	0.542	0.700	0.879	1.093	1.372	1.812	2.228	2.764	3.169	4.587
11	0.129	0.260	0.396	0.540	0.697	0.876	1.088	1.363	1.796	2.201	2.718	3.106	4.437
12	0.128	0.259	0.395	0.539	0.695	0.873	1.083	1.356	1.782	2.179	2.681	3.055	4.318
13	0.128	0.259	0.394	0.538	0.694	0.870	1.079	1.350	1.771	2.160	2.650	3.012	4.221
14	0.128	0.258	0.393	0.537	0.692	0.868	1.076	1.345	1.761	2.145	2.624	2.977	4.140
15	0.128	0.258	0.393	0.536	0.691	0.866	1.074	1.341	1.753	2.131	2.602	2.947	4.073
16	0.128	0.258	0.392	0.535	0.690	0.865	1.071	1.337	1.746	2.120	2.583	2.921	4.015
17	0.128	0.257	0.392	0.534	0.689	0.863	1.069	1.333	1.74	2.110	2.567	2.898	3.965
18	0.127	0.257	0.392	0.534	0.688	0.862	1.067	1.330	1.734	2.101	2.552	2.878	3.922
19	0.127	0.257	0.391	0.533	0.688	0.861	1.066	1.328	1.729	2.093	2.539	2.861	3.883
20	0.127	0.257	0.391	0.533	0.687	0.86	1.064	1.325	1.725	2.086	2.528	2.845	3.850
21	0.127	0.257	0.391	0.532	0.686	0.859	1.063	1.323	1.721	2.080	2.518	2.831	3.819
22	0.127	0.256	0.390	0.532	0.686	0.858	1.061	1.321	1.717	2.074	2.508	2.819	3.792

contd...

n	0.90	0.80	0.70	0.60	0.50	0.40	0.30	0.20	0.10	0.05	0.02	0.01	0.001
23	0.127	0.256	0.390	0.532	0.685	0.858	1.060	1.319	1.714	2.069	2.500	2.807	3.767
24	0.127	0.256	0.390	0.531	0.685	0.857	1.059	1.318	1.711	2.064	2.492	2.797	3.745
25	0.127	0.256	0.390	0.531	0.684	0.856	1.058	1.316	1.708	2.060	2.485	2.787	3.725
26	0.127	0.256	0.390	0.531	0.684	0.856	1.058	1.315	1.706	2.056	2.479	2.779	3.707
27	0.127	0.256	0.389	0.531	0.684	0.855	1.057	1.314	1.703	2.052	2.473	2.771	3.690
28	0.127	0.256	0.389	0.53	0.683	0.855	1.056	1.313	1.701	2.048	2.467	2.763	3.674
29	0.127	0.256	0.389	0.53	0.683	0.854	1.055	1.311	1.699	2.045	2.462	2.756	3.659
30	0.127	0.256	0.389	0.53	0.683	0.854	1.055	1.310	1.697	2.042	2.457	2.75	3.646
40	0.126	0.255	0.388	0.529	0.681	0.851	1.05	1.303	1.684	2.021	2.423	2.704	3.551
60	0.126	0.254	0.387	0.527	0.679	0.848	1.046	1.296	1.671	2.000	2.300	2.660	3.460
120	0.126	0.254	0.386	0.526	0.677	0.845	1.041	1.289	1.658	1.980	2.358	2.617	3.373
00	0.126	0.253	0.385	0.524	0.674	0.842	1.036	1.282	1.645	1.060	2.326	2.576	3.201

Appendix 4: Table of χ^2 distribution

N	0.99	0.98	0.95	0.9	0.8	0.7	0.5	0.3	0.2	0.1	0.05	0.02	0.01	0.001
1	0.0002	0.0063	0.0039	0.016	0.064	0.148	0.455	1.074	1.642	2.706	3.841	5.412	6.635	10.827
2	0.0201	0.0404	0.103	0.211	0.446	0.713	1.386	2.408	3.219	4.605	5.991	7.824	9.21	13.815
3	0.115	0.185	0.352	0.584	1.005	1.424	2.366	3.665	4.642	6.251	7.815	9.837	11.345	16.266
4	0.297	0.429	0.711	1.064	1.649	2.195	3.357	4.878	5.989	7.779	9.488	11.668	13.277	18.467
5	0.554	0.752	1.145	1.610	2.343	3.000	4.351	6.064	7.289	9.236	11.070	13.388	15.086	20.515
6	0.872	1.134	1.635	2.204	3.070	3.828	5.348	7.231	8.558	10.645	12.592	15.033	16.812	22.457
7	1.239	1.564	2.167	2.833	3.822	4.671	6.346	8.383	9.803	12.017	14.067	16.622	18.475	24.322
8	1.646	2.032	2.733	3.490	4.594	5.527	7.344	9.524	11.030	13.362	15.507	18.168	20.090	26.125
9	2.088	2.532	3.325	4.168	5.380	6.393	8.343	10.656	12.242	14.684	16.919	19.679	21.666	27.877
10	2.558	3.059	3.940	4.865	6.179	7.267	9.342	11.781	13.442	15.987	18.307	21.161	23.209	29.588
11	3.053	3.609	4.575	5.578	6.989	8.148	10.341	12.899	14.631	17.275	19.675	22.618	24.725	31.264
12	3.571	4.178	5.226	6.304	7.807	9.034	11.340	14.011	15.812	18.549	21.026	24.054	26.217	32.909
13	4.107	4.765	5.892	7.042	8.634	9.926	12.340	15.119	16.985	19.812	22.362	25.472	27.688	34.528
14	4.660	5.368	6.571	7.790	9.467	10.821	13.339	16.222	18.151	21.064	23.685	26.873	29.141	36.123
15	5.229	5.985	7.261	8.547	10.307	11.721	14.339	17.322	19.311	22.307	24.996	28.259	30.578	37.697
16	5.812	6.614	7.962	9.312	11.152	12.624	15.338	18.418	20.465	23.542	26.296	29.633	32.000	39.252
17	6.408	7.255	8.672	10.085	12.002	13.531	15.338	19.511	21.615	24.769	27.587	30.995	33.409	40.790
18	7.015	7.906	9.390	10.865	12.857	14.440	17.338	20.601	22.760	25.989	28.869	32.346	34.805	42.312
19	7.633	8.567	10.117	11.651	13.716	15.352	18.338	21.689	23.900	27.204	30.144	33.687	36.191	43.820
20	8.260	9.237	10.851	12.443	14.578	16.266	19.337	22.775	25.038	28.412	31.410	35.020	37.566	45.315
21	8.897	9.915	11.591	13.240	15.445	17.182	20.337	23.858	26.171	29.615	32.671	36.343	38.932	46.797
22	9.542	10.600	12.338	14.041	16.314	18.101	21.337	24.939	27.301	30.813	33.924	37.659	40.289	48.268
23	10.196	11.293	13.091	14.848	17.187	19.021	22.337	26.018	28.429	32.007	35.172	38.968	41.638	49.782
24	10.856	11.992	13.848	15.659	18.062	19.943	23.337	27.096	29.553	33.196	36.415	40.270	42.980	51.179
25	11.524	12.697	14.611	16.473	18.940	20.867	24.337	28.172	30. 675	34.382	37.652	41.566	44.314	52.620

contd...

N	0.99	0.98	0.95	0.9	0.8	0.7	0.5	0.3	0.2	0.1	0.05	0.02	0.01	0.001
26	12.198	13.409	15.379	17.292	19.820	21.792	25.336	29.246	31.795	35.563	38.885	42.856	45.642	54.052
27	12.879	14.125	16.151	18.114	20.703	22.719	26.336	30.319	32.912	36.741	40.113	44.140	46.963	55.476
28	13.565	14.847	16.928	18.939	21.588	23.647	27.336	31.391	34.027	37.916	41.337	45.419	48.278	56.893
29	14.256	15.574	17.708	19.768	22.475	24.577	28.336	32.461	35.139	39.087	42.557	46.693	49.588	58.302
30	14.953	16.306	18.493	20.599	23.364	25.508	29.336	33.530	36.250	40.256	43.773	47.962	50.892	59.703
32	16.362	17.783	20.072	22.271	25.148	27.373	31.336	35.665	38.466	42.585	46.194	50.487	53.486	62.487
34	17.789	19.275	21.664	23.952	26.938	29.242	33.336	37.795	40.676	44.903	48.602	52.995	56.061	65.247
36	19.233	20.783	23.269	25.643	28.735	31.115	35.336	39.922	42.879	47.212	50.999	55.489	58.619	67.985
38	20.691	22.304	24.884	27.343	30.537	32.992	37.335	42.045	45.076	49.513	53.384	57.969	61.162	70.703
40	22.164	23.838	26.509	29.051	32.345	34.872	39.335	44.165	47.269	51.805	55.759	60.436	63.691	73.402
42	23.650	25.383	28.144	30.765	34.157	36.755	41.335	46.282	49.456	54.090	58.124	62.892	66.206	76.084
44	25.148	26.939	29.787	32.487	35.974	38.641	43.335	48.396	51.639	56.369	60.481	65.337	68.710	78.750
46	26.657	28.504	31.439	34.215	37.795	40.529	45.335	50.507	53.818	58.641	62.830	67.771	71.201	81.400
48	28.177	30.080	33.098	35.949	39.621	42.420	47.335	52.616	55.993	60.907	65.171	70.197	73.683	84.037
50	29.707	31.664	34.764	37.689	41.449	44.313	49.335	54.723	58.164	63.167	67.505	72.613	76.154	86.661
52	31.246	33.256	36.437	39.433	43.281	46.209	51.335	56.827	60.332	65.422	69.832	75.021	78.616	89.272
54	32.793	34.856	38.116	41.183	45.117	48.106	53.335	58.930	62.496	67.673	72.153	7.4220	81.069	91.872
56	34.350	36.464	39.801	42.937	46.955	50.005	55.335	61.031	64.658	69.919	74.468	79.815	83.513	94.461
58	35.913	38.078	41.492	44.696	48.797	51.906	57.335	63.129	66.816	72.160	76.778	82.201	85.950	97.039
60	37.485	39.699	43.188	46.459	50.641	53.809	59.335	65.227	68.972	74.397	79.082	84.580	88.379	99.607
62	39.063	41.327	44.889	48.226	52.487	55.714	61.335	67.322	71.125	76.630	81.381	86.953	90.802	102.166
64	40.649	42.960	46.595	49.996	54.336	57.620	63.335	69.416	73.276	78.860	83.675	89.320	93.217	104.716
66	42.240	44.599	48.305	51.770	56.188	59.527	65.335	71.508	75.424	81.085	85.965	91.681	95.626	107.258
68	43.838	46.244	50.020	53.548	58.042	61.436	67.335	73.600	77.571	83.308	88.250	94.037	98.028	109.791
70	45.442	47.893	51.739	55.329	59.898	63.346	69.334	75.689	79.715	85.527	90.531	96.388	100.425	112.317

Appendix 5: Table of normal distribution

P	0.00	0.01	0.02	0.03	0.04	0.05	0.06	0.07	0.08	0.09
0.0	∞	2.575829	2.326348	2.170090	2.053749	1.959964	1.880794	1.811911	1.750686	1.695398
0.1	1.644854	1.598193	1.554774	1.514102	1.475791	1.439531	1.405072	1.372204	1.340755	1.310579
0.2	1.281552	1.253565	1.226528	1.200359	1.174987	1.150349	1.126391	1.103063	1.080319	1.058122
0.3	1.036433	1.015222	0.994458	0.974114	0.954165	0.934589	0.915365	0.896473	0.877896	0.859617
0.4	0.841621	0.823894	0.806421	0.789192	0.772193	0.755415	0.738847	0.722479	0.706303	0.690309
0.5	0.674490	0.658838	0.643345	0.628006	0.612813	0.597760	0.582842	0.568051	0.553385	0.538836
0.6	0.524401	0.510073	0.495850	0.481727	0.467699	0.453762	0.439913	0.426148	0.412463	0.398855
0.7	0.385320	0.371856	0.358459	0.345126	0.331853	0.318639	0.305481	0.292375	0.279319	0.266311
0.8	0.253347	0.240426	0.227545	0.214702	0.201893	0.189118	0.176374	0.163658	0.150969	0.138304
0.9	0.125661	0.113039	0.100434	0.087845	0.075270	0.062707	0.050154	0.037608	0.025069	0.012533

P	0.002	0.001	0.000,1	0.000,01	0.000,001	0.000,000,1	0.000,000,01	0.000,000,001
x	3.09023	3.29053	3.89059	4.14717	4.89164	5.32672	5.73073	6.10941

The value of P for each entry is found by adding the column heading to the value in the left hand margin. The corresponding value of x is the deviation such that the probability of an observation falling outside the range - x to +x is P. For example P = 0.03 for x = 2.170090; so that 3 percent of normally distributed values will have positive or negative deviations exceeding the standard deviation in the ratio 2.170090 at least.

Appendix 6: Table of T-values for Wilcoxon's signed rank test

Number of pairs	P = 0.05	P = 0.01
7	2	0
8	2	0
9	6	2
10	8	3
11	11	5
12	14	7
13	17	10
14	21	13
15	25	16
16	29	19

Values of *T*, equal or smaller than the above indicate rejection of the null hypothesis

Appendix 7: Table of T-values at 5 per cent level for Mann-Whitney test

n_1 → n_2 ↓	2	3	4	5	6	7	8	9	10	11	12	13	14	15
4			10											
5		6	11	17										
6		7	12	18	26									
7		7	13	20	27	36								
8	3	8	14	21	29	38	49							
9	3	8	15	22	31	40	51	63						
10	3	9	15	23	32	42	53	65	78					
11	4	9	16	24	34	44	55	68	81	96				
12	4	10	17	26	35	46	58	71	85	99	115			
13	4	10	18	27	37	48	60	73	88	103	119	137		
14	4	11	19	28	38	50	63	76	91	106	123	141	160	
15	4	11	20	29	40	52	65	79	94	110	127	145	164	185
16	4	12	21	31	42	54	67	82	97	114	131	150	169	
17	5	12	21	32	43	56	70	84	100	117	135	154		
18	5	13	22	33	45	58	72	87	103	121	139			
19	5	13	23	34	46	60	74	90	107	124				
20	5	14	24	35	48	62	77	93	110					
21	6	14	25	37	50	64	79	95						
22	6	15	26	38	51	66	82							
23	6	15	27	39	53	68								
24	6	16	28	40	55									
25	6	16	28	42										
26	7	17	29											
27	7	17												
28	7													

n_1 and n_2 are the number of cases in the two groups. When the groups are of unequal size n_1 refers to the smaller.

Values equal or smaller than the tabulated values causes rejection of the null hypothesis.

Index

E

F

G

H

L

M

N